The Best You

The B

Through

Hypnosis

Total Mind and Body Transformation

Cristina Di Nardo-Dupre, MSW, LICSW

The Best You Through Hypnosis

The Best You Through Hypnosis

The Best You Through Hypnosis:
Total Mind and Body Transformation / Cristina Di Nardo-Dupre

ISBN 978-0-692-33106-4

1. Health   2. Weight Loss   3. Diet   4. Nutrition

Editors: Liz Kibby and MP Barker
Cover: JR Photography and H. Noelle
Layout: Meghan Bachand
Consultants: Emily Kravetz

For more information about The Best You Through Hypnosis and Cristina's program, please visit **www.thebestyouthroughhypnosis.com** or call **413-789-9198.**

Dedication

This book is dedicated to my beautiful parents, who taught me all about nutrition as I was growing up in Italy. It is also dedicated to you, dear reader, and to those who are searching for a healthy lifestyle in this contemporary and busy world.

Disclaimer

The information provided in this book is intended only to be used for educational purposes on the subjects discussed. This book is sold with an understanding that it is not meant to be, nor should it be used, to provide medical advice of any kind, including but not limited to diagnosing, prescribing, or treating any disease, condition, illness, or injury. The publisher and author are not responsible for any health or allergy needs that may require medical supervision and are not liable for any damages or negative consequences for any action or application of this book to any person reading or following the information herein. It is essential that before beginning any diet or exercise program, including any aspect of this book, each individual consults a licensed physician for a full medical clearance. References are provided for informational purposes only and do not constitute endorsement of any products or other sources. Readers should be aware that the websites listed in this book may change.

The audio files provided on our website are not to be listened to while operating a motor vehicle or other heavy machinery or equipment. The author and publisher claim no responsibility to any person or entity for any liability, loss, or damage caused or alleged to be caused directly or indirectly as a result of any use, application, or interpretation of this book and the materials included.

Table of Contents

The Best You Through Hypnosis

Acknowledgements

A special thanks goes to my granddaughter Elizabeth Kibby, for her countless time and support on editing the book, sampling food with me, making, taking pictures of, and enjoying these recipes.

The book was developed with the help of my office manager, Meghan Bachand, when we first began seeing great results on weight loss through our program. We thought, *"Wouldn't it be great if we could reach people throughout the United States and eventually the whole world by writing a book with a complete plan through recipes and a healthy lifestyle."* We found that other books and recipes always include nuts, starch, and sugar, which we omit during the period of weight loss in our eating plan. The only choice we had was to write our own and make it available to everyone. Even though this idea sprang to our minds six years ago, it never came to fruition until now because we wanted to make sure the program was successful long term.

As I was managing my private practice by seeing clients for counseling as well as running my Weight Loss through Hypnosis group, I realized I needed to find someone who has the same interests that I have and is in the field of social work like me. I searched around at different colleges and was blessed to have found my answer at Springfield College. They sent Emily Kravetz, a student completing her final year of graduate school in the Master of Social Work program and who plans to get her master's in nutrition. It seemed to be a perfect match. Not only has she been able to get experience on her case and group work for her college requirements, but she is getting experience by running the weight loss group, gathering research information, and validating progress through research. When I would have ideas, she was able to bring them to life through her great writing skills.

One day I said to my husband, Charles J. Dupre, "I am thinking of writing a book on healthy lifestyle." His response, "Oh no, don't think, because when you think of something, you have already created it!" And he was right! His fear was that I would spend long days and late nights working on the book; however, he has always understood my work. A special thanks goes to him for his constant moral support, as well as tremendous financial support.

The true driving force on authoring this book began several years ago when Mary Lou Di Giacomo and her cousin Linda were telling me, "You need to write that book!" I remember saying, "But English is my second language. I don't know if I could do it." They told me, "Don't worry, just put your ideas down and we will help you polish the English." We even thought of a title--*Contemporary Approach to a Healthy Lifestyle through Hypnosis*--although we did not end up using it due to the length. With their encouragement, I did start writing my ideas down. Every few weeks, Mary Lou would call me to make sure I was continuing to work on the book. I thank them for not giving up on me.

Foreword

It has been one of the greatest joys I have experienced to be able to help my grandmother, Cristina, write this book.

We have taken the program she has spent years developing and perfecting and put it into words. We even took it one step further to give you these simple recipes that will have you feeling confident and comfortable in the kitchen from now on.

Although the program began with weight loss in mind, I firmly believe that anyone of any size can benefit from following the program outlined here. As a former anorexic, I can tell you that being part of the program taught me how to understand the relationship between my mind and body in a way I did not know before. It helped me get into the kitchen and learn how to cook and eat nutritionally for my body. It even helped me to eliminate the fear of going into a restaurant and upsetting the staff with special requests, something I was not comfortable doing before.

Cristina is not the first, nor the only person to use hypnosis to help others to achieve a healthy lifestyle. I have witnessed many of her clients come to her after having previously gone to another program and gotten only short-term results.

The people who come to her program find long-term success because she goes above and beyond to ensure each of her clients understands how to maintain a healthy lifestyle through total mind and body integration. She teaches and empowers you to take your healthy lifestyle out of her office and integrate it into the real world, which is where so many of us meet health challenges. Also, Cristina always stays in touch with her former clients, offering refreshers and ongoing support.

I thank you for choosing this book to help you find the best version of yourself. As you read this book, you are taking the first step towards a healthy lifestyle; you are supporting a woman who deserves recognition for being such a giving and hardworking person. She gives without thinking of what she can get in return. She has my admiration and, after reading this book, I am confident she will have yours, too.

Liz Kibby

Preface

A Word from Cristina

When I came to the United States from Italy in 1968, I remember being a size four. I was never worried about my weight or what I ate, because in Italy we ate healthy and we were active, so this was not a concern. We did not eat processed food, canned food, or foods with preservatives. We most definitely did not eat cake or sweets on a daily basis. However, we did eat fruit that was in season.

I did not think to be concerned with my size, but after a month in the United States my friends began to tell me, "Cristina! You are gaining weight!" I remember I told them that it meant I was healthy, because my mom always said, "Being healthy doesn't mean skinny, it means well built." However, I soon came to realize that after only a month I had gained about fifteen pounds. That's when I became aware that I did, in fact, have a problem. My friends and I were all eating processed foods, chips, cake, and sweets for most meals, so I thought, "Well, maybe that's just the way they eat in the United States, so I can't change things."

As my understanding of the culture improved over time, I began to notice that people who wanted to lose weight or keep it off, went to the gym. But this was only one part of the solution; exercise was not the total answer. I observed a cycle that would repeat itself: exercise in the morning, eating and drinking to excess at night, and starting all over again the next day. It was becoming clear to me that physical activity did not negate the effects of unhealthy eating and drinking. In spite of this, I would go to the gym every day and try to keep my size down to a four to six. However, I was always in fear of gaining weight.

I continued in this pattern for a number of years, until my work became such a priority that I could no longer make time to go to the gym. It was then that I decided to conduct research to find answers to this cultural phenomenon. "Can I eat healthy in this busy and contemporary world as well as be fit without spending all my time at the gym?" The question boggled my mind.

Through my reading I found that Mark Sisson and Jennifer Meier had authored several books based on the "*Primal Blueprint*." These guides explained how our ancestors were able to eat healthy and stay fit during the time of hunter-gatherers, and how we can take steps to take advantage of the evolutionary tools that have been passed down to our modern generation.

I found myself inspired that there were others like me out there, seeking a solution to our common problem. While exploring this lifestyle, I came to the realization that this simple way of living was exactly how my parents, in Italy, had taken care of our family, through healthy nutrition and plenty of physical activity. Determined to share this newfound hope to become healthy again with others, I set off to spread the word. Although I didn't know it at the time, I believed that this could become a reality. I continued to nurture the idea of writing a book which you now hold in your hands, and it will be a guide for you in your new healthy lifestyle.

-Cristina Di Nardo-Dupre, MSW, LICSW

Introduction

This program is 99% successful for those who implement it, whether in groups or individually, and may use refreshers as needed. If you are tired of the "yo-yo" dieting trap, feeling as though you can never lose the weight and keep it off, then this book is for you. With the aid of recipes, a daily outline to follow and the hypnosis that I have spent years developing, you will find an entirely new approach to building a sound mind and healthy body.

When I started this program 14 years ago, my clients had so many questions. Nine years ago, I decided to write this book to help my clients navigate the program. I have worked with thousands of clients to help them to reach their lifestyle goals since then. Based on feedback from my clients, 99% feel that they have acquired a power over their body that they did not have before.

My clients believe that this book makes the program so easy to follow and keeps them motivated. The magic of clinical hypnosis is able to touch their subconscious and when combined with Cognitive Behavioral Theory, food is no longer an obsession, and they have no desire to eat junk food. Following the six incentives has made it possible for so many to reach their goals and maintain a healthy lifestyle.

During the Covid-19 pandemic, I stopped seeing groups to keep my clients safe. I was only seeing individuals or couples for quite a while. While I have resumed groups now, I learned that by doing the hypnosis stage of the session separately, I was able to customize and support my clients and their needs in a better way. I believe that the program is successful individually or in a group, but I will perform the clinical hypnosis part separately going forward.

My clients are doing very well, and refreshers aren't needed as much. In the past, after the three sessions, I was scheduling a refresher within a month and since I have been doing the hypnosis component separately, I have noticed a decrease in the need for the refresher. Of course, things happen in life and some traumatic events can make clients feel out of control and that's when my refreshers are needed.

I believe that this book is the ultimate tool for clients doing in-person sessions and have found that with the help of PowerPoint and Zoom, I can reach and help clients further away. I need to be able to see the clients' face during the hypnosis portion of the program to be effective and feel connected.

My clients have changed their view of what food means for them. Before they were part of this large group that were accustomed to yo-yo dieting and would reward themselves with unhealthy food once they had been eating healthy for a while. Through the Cognitive Behavioral Theory and Hypnosis, my clients have been able to develop a consistent way to eat healthy by choosing the right foods and feeling strong and satisfied with their new healthy lifestyle. This gave my clients the power to control what they can eat and what they cannot eat. It is not up to their body anymore, but their mind. The change comes from inside and changes the clients' core beliefs about food and health.

The History of this Book

In my last thirty-five years working as a Licensed Independent Clinical Social Worker in the field of mental health, I have discovered when working with children, families, and couples, that there is a great need to help people who are going through difficulties in their lives. Individuals quite often have difficulty achieving their aspirations and goals.

In light of this knowledge, I have increased my training from counseling outward, into the fields of spirituality, hypnosis, relaxation, and desensitization. Developing the ability to connect the mind and the body is very powerful, but unfortunately not widely integrated yet in modern society.

I have studied and researched many types of compulsive eating behaviors. I have tried to understand how this symptom shows up so strongly in those who are unable to make that mind-body connection due to trauma or other circumstances in their lives. Personally, I have been seeking to discover how I could help people change their food perceptions. I have witnessed clients who starve themselves, overeat, or only eat at night and I have very much wanted to help them not only to overcome the unhealthy behaviors, but also to replace those actions with new healthy eating habits.

On the other hand, people have sought my help who usually eat healthy, but find themselves overwhelmed by cravings for sugar or starch, particularly in the evenings and on weekends. Boredom, stress, loss, or other uncontrollable emotions lead them to continue to eat unhealthy, gain weight, and follow the vicious cycle of unhealthy eating. The development of these harmful

9

eating habits brings people to a stuck position and, at times, to feelings of panic when they are unable to see the way out.

I have used hypnotherapy, guided imagery, and relaxation to help my clients overcome maladies such as fear, anxiety, panic, trauma, nightmares, sleepwalking, and smoking cessation. In the past sixteen years, I have discovered that by combining hypnosis with Cognitive Behavioral Theory, harmful eating behaviors can also be removed and replaced by healthy eating patterns.

In my work, I've found Cognitive Behavioral Theory can be easily explained and understood as the geometric shape of a triangle, with the three points labeled to reflect the three ways we process information: Thinking, Action, and Feeling. **(Figure 1)** By looking at the red arrow in the triangle, we can see that once a cycle of negative thinking begins, it is hard to break. The negative thinking brings negative actions by eating the unhealthy food again. After eating unhealthy food, you feel upset, fat, miserable and trapped and now you go back to your negative thinking and feelings. They feed each other, like a vicious cycle. Sometimes the vicious cycle becomes so intense, people will go into panic. We understand that it is difficult to change our feelings unless we change our thinking and our actions as well.

Figure 1

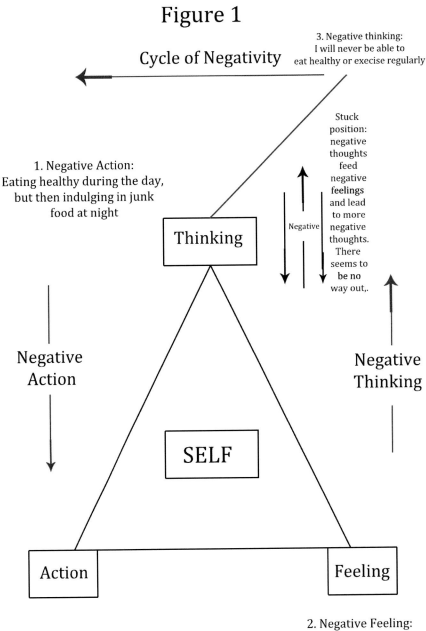

Cycle of Negativity

3. Negative thinking:
I will never be able to
eat healthy or exercise regularly

1. Negative Action:
Eating healthy during the day,
but then indulging in junk
food at night

Thinking

Stuck
position:
negative
thoughts
feed
negative
feelings
and lead
Negative   to more
negative
thoughts.
There
seems to
be no
way out,.

Negative
Action

Negative
Thinking

SELF

Action

Feeling

2. Negative Feeling:
I feel bloated, ugly and
unyhappy

Negative Feelings

Figure 2

Cycle of Positivity

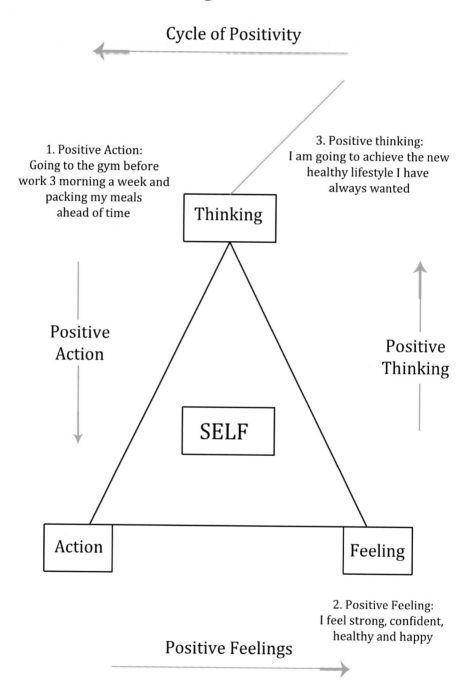

1. Positive Action: Going to the gym before work 3 morning a week and packing my meals ahead of time

3. Positive thinking: I am going to achieve the new healthy lifestyle I have always wanted

Thinking

Positive Action

Positive Thinking

SELF

Action

Feeling

2. Positive Feeling: I feel strong, confident, healthy and happy

Positive Feelings

In Figure 2., marked with a green arrow – a person is able to come out of the negative cycle by visualizing a new healthy lifestyle. This is done by following the six incentives with meal preparation, eating protein and vegetables, doing exercises, creating a positive sense of self, developing healthy habits, and listening to the hypnosis recording daily. You will continue to visualize the size you want to be and follow the six incentives necessary to achieve your goal. As you follow, you are able to actualize your goal by doing it. Now that you have created consistency between your thinking and your actions, the result is going to be a positive one by feeling healthy, energetic, happy, and free. In conclusion, the only way that you can break the negative cycle is by creating a new way of thinking and action, rather than remaining stuck on the negative feelings.

Deeper Explanation of the Negative and Positive Cycle

Imagine coming home from a stressful day at work, and having the need to eat something that you believe will make you feel better. You turn to sweets, chips, or junk food that will give you an immediate response of relief or pleasure in the body and mind. In the long run, this has not fixed your problem. When you eat the wrong foods, you feel guilty and angry with yourself once the immediate satisfaction wears off, and you realize that the bad feelings are still somehow there. So, you eat again to subdue them for just a moment, and the negative cycle continues without pause.

Assuming you have the same stressful day as before, but this time, you decide you can take a different course of action by changing the insidious negative thoughts into more positive ones. This time instead of reaching for unhealthy food, you take the initiative to perform a healthy action. This could be taking a walk, reading a good book, talking with your friends, or doing anything else that would make you feel good about yourself. All of these actions bring positive results that will connect your mind to realizing the goal you had, which was to feel better after a long day at work.

You can see that once you've changed your thoughts through your actions, you have thus changed your feelings, and all three parts of the triangle now come together harmoniously. This is the beginning of a new positive cycle, but you must continue to visualize this healthier behavior to truly implement the positive cycle into your life. Focusing on what is healthy--such as exercise, painting, hobbies, eating healthy for your body, and repeating positive affirmations throughout the day — are ways to help you develop new positive behaviors so you can begin to feel in harmony with yourself and the world around you.

The Purpose of this Book

The purpose of this book is to give you the confidence to love your body, be the size you want to be and maintain it and let go of the fear of gaining weight.

I would love to personally be able to help each individual learn how to love their body, feel comfortable in it, and have the ability to make healthy choices so they can let go of the fear of gaining weight. However, even the barriers of distance can be broken because through this book you will be receiving exactly the same treatment my clients receive at my office. Cristina also offers her program via online sessions. If you are interested, please contact our office to book these sessions. This book will help you follow our program step by step. Those who are currently participating or have already participated in the program with me at my Center and wish to have more information and instruction about which foods to eat and how to prepare them will find this book very useful.

Through the years, while conducting sessions with my clients, many tend to ask the same questions about food, time after time. Frequently, they ask what kind of condiments can be used on their food or to marinate meat and vegetables due to the fact that most bottled sauces generally are processed and unhealthy. The majority of the condiments, dressings, and marinades sold on the shelves contain MSG (monosodium glutamate) as well as artificial sweeteners such as sucralose, aspartame, and others. My clients have also wanted to know what kinds of foods are considered processed and what foods would be wholesome and natural alternatives.

I have found that during sessions I am always being asked about what recipes to use. Although a number are provided on my

15

website, I realized that if my clients had a cookbook to follow, they would be able to spend less time researching and more time actually cooking and enjoying their meals. It is my desire to make the program simple and easy to follow in order to produce the most change towards a healthy lifestyle.

The recipes in this book are written in a very straightforward way. I use natural, unprocessed foods just as they were used for many years in my old country, Italy. Some of these recipes were shown to me by my mom when I was as young as thirteen or fourteen years old. At that age, I was preparing these meals myself, so it should be simple for you to now replicate the recipes presented.

A Method That Works

This book was originally written to answer the continual requests of my clients in my program entitled "Weight Loss through Hypnosis." The program is attended at my office for a total of three sessions, with optional refresher sessions afterward. Sessions usually last around an hour and a half for individuals and two hours for a group.

In the first session, I learn about each person's experience with weight loss and what has and hasn't worked. Then, I explain the difference between other weight loss programs and our program. Our program is different because we do not use any prepackaged diet foods that are usually high in sodium and contain additives that create toxins in your body. We eat only wholesome food which means it is unaltered from its original or natural state; not processed. For more information, please see our food list on page 36. I explain the difference on how we monitor our progress, by omitting the scale and visualizing the self by eating healthy and exercising. The emphasis is not on the weight like other programs, but it is on the size that the person wants to reach. By eating protein, a person will build muscle which is heavier than fat therefore we encourage people to use measurements rather than weight. More will be explained on page 24. I provide all the information such as, list of foods and recommended vitamins. I explain the Six Incentives (tools) in detail as well as the Cognitive Behavioral Theory. At the end of the session, I explain what hypnosis is and how it works. After the hypnosis, everyone feels relaxed, positive, and ready to begin a new healthy lifestyle. In order for the process to continue, the hypnosis recording is emailed to each person. A hypnosis recording to help them to sleep is also emailed if they choose.

After a week, people meet for the second session to reinforce what has been taught in the first and to expand upon it. People are able to express feelings, progress, difficulties as well as exchange information on cooking and recipes. Hypnosis is administered again at the end of this session.

The third session is two weeks after the second. By this time people feel that they have mastered the program. That means they have learned how to let go of the cravings, develop new healthy habits, and they are on their way to reaching their goal. Also, a plan of action is developed to follow after they reach their goal.

The program is geared towards individuals who are highly motivated to succeed and ready to follow the step-by-step process as outlined in this book. Cristina does offer this program in the office to small groups.

One last crucial note before you begin, we strongly advise that you first consult a physician before applying any information found in this book. If you are taking medication, it is crucial that you talk to your doctor to be medically cleared before embarking on this journey. Your medical condition may change drastically as your new healthy lifestyle will change your body very quickly if the program is followed the way I explain it. This applies especially to those taking insulin, as this medication will need to be reduced with a physician's permission.

We are eager to hear about your success as you follow along, and your experience will aid us to continue evolving our program to help you be as successful as possible. We are happy to hear from you by emailing **duprehypnosis@gmail.com** or calling our office at (413) 789-9198. You can find more information to guide your journey to a healthy lifestyle on our website:

www.thebestyouthroughhypnosis.com

Truth vs. Misconception about Hypnosis

Sometimes people have acquired the wrong idea about how hypnosis works. Some people believe that someone can put wrong ideas into their mind or make them do things that they do not want to. Others believe that it does not work. All of these preconceived ideas are learned through movies and TV and are inaccurate. When clinical hypnosis is used appropriately, with a person you trust, it can produce powerful life changes. Hypnotic suggestion only works in congruence with the person's beliefs. People already come with the intention or want to have a healthy lifestyle. The information I am giving during the hypnosis is the same as what the person absorbed during the sessions, just reinforced in a deeper level so they remain in the subconscious mind. Research has shown that at least 89% of people are able to go into a deep trance. Yes, everyone can be hypnotized if they choose to. Hypnosis, relaxation, and visualization are very powerful tools to overcome cravings and unhealthy habits. The initial stage of hypnosis focuses on helping the person to achieve total body relaxation. The mind during the hypnosis is able to absorb 90% of what has been said and has the ability to retain it. The mind will then release it in daily life. For example, if a person picks up a soda to drink it, the subconscious immediately comes in and tells the person that they cannot have that. When this happens over and over, it becomes a healthy choice instead of an unhealthy habit. During the hypnosis, the person has the power to let go of sweets, starch and alcohol or may choose to hold onto one of these. If that is the case, the person will struggle later to let go of it. The most important factor for success is measured by the drive a person has to reach their goal. If they choose to let go, they will find this healthy lifestyle is very easy to follow.

A Fresh Start

Prior to my decision to write this book with these specific recipes, I researched everywhere for any other books written like this that integrate a healthy lifestyle through the tool of hypnosis. Although the concepts and methods outlined have been around for a long time, I have never seen integrating them together.

At the beginning of the program, my clients cut out certain foods which include sweets, starches, grains, and fruits, from their eating plan until their goal is reached. However, unlike other eating styles, we reintroduce most of these foods to the diet after the goal size has been achieved. The only things that are never brought back are the very processed foods that are so unhealthy in any amount. I can be sure to tell you that after following the program for a week or two you will not miss those nutritionally lacking foods.

The Program

By working with this program, you will learn to find a positive balance in your life by preparing your healthy meals ahead of time, enjoying your physical exercise, repeating positive affirmations to yourself, and focusing on what is healthy for you and dropping what is unhealthy. When I say "healthy," I want you to know it doesn't always mean just the food you eat, but also the positive energy you will be sending to yourself and others.

I truly believe that each one of us has the potential and ability to live the life we dream of when we connect the unconscious with the conscious mind. Great things can happen for all of us when both parts are in harmony. Our mind has a great ability to visualize what the body alone cannot conceive. Through visualization, all of us can break barriers and heal our injured selves, as well as achieve personal goals.

It is a known fact that our unconscious mind is responsible for the majority of the learning our brain does. Logically, we must have access to that part of our brain if we are to make the meaningful lifestyle changes, we have just discussed. As I stated before, hypnosis and relaxation, when administered correctly by a person you trust, are tools that can produce powerful life changes.

Each person who elects to be hypnotized has full control of their mind throughout but makes a conscious decision to relax the body. Thus, in relaxation the mind is ready to fully absorb what is being said by myself through hypnosis.

You may find yourself excited and eager to begin this program by the prospect of such positive changes in your life. I, too, am excited for you to discover your new healthy lifestyle but remember: the most important factor for success in this program is measured by the drive and motivation of each individual to succeed.

You will be learning a whole new way of acting and thinking about life, and it may not always be easy to do so until you begin to reap the rewards of your labor. The hypnosis will help you along this journey to the extent you let it. So just relax, feel proud that you've already taken the first positive actions towards growth, and we will move forward together toward health and happiness.

How It Works – Cristina's Six Incentives

Weight Loss through Hypnosis is a program that teaches you how to live a healthy lifestyle over a period of three weeks. Once you have learned the tools, you will continue with it until you reach your goal. There are six tools, or incentives, we use in order to reach your goal. In this program, your goal will be the size you wish to achieve. I will urge you to throw out your scale and stop worrying about pounds.

During our first session together, I ask my clients what their current clothing size is, and what size they would like to be. In this way, we remove the obsession of counting calories and constantly stepping on the scale and make it easy to notice how the program is working. Measuring yourself is an option, if desired; however, you will find that through this program it is the way your body feels, how your clothes fit, and the ways in which your mind will adapt to a healthy way of living that are far more important in measuring success.

The six incentives I mentioned are:

1.   Prepare your meals in advance.

2.   Follow the meal plan by eating protein with equal amounts of vegetables.

3.   Exercise at least three times a week.

4.   Develop a positive sense of self.

5.   Create new positive eating habits.

6.   Listen to the hypnosis recording daily.

First Incentive:
Prepare your meals in advance

The first incentive, along with this book, will teach you how to prepare your meals in advance. I know most of us would love to have the time to prepare each meal fresh, as they did in the old country. Unfortunately, our contemporary lifestyle does not give us that luxury, so through the program we are going to learn to make large quantities of healthy food in advance and freeze or store them until ready to eat. Typically, more time is spent preparing dinner, so we focus on learning how to prepare healthy breakfasts, lunches, and snacks in advance. This way, rather than reaching for easy, processed foods that are so prevalent in today's modern, busy world, we will find ourselves with wholesome, delightfully natural food to indulge in at each mealtime.

<u>Second Incentive:</u>
Follow the meal plan given to you

The second incentive is easy to follow and consists of eating a balanced diet of protein with an equal, or slightly smaller, amount of vegetables. Protein provides our amino acids, which break down the starch and sugar naturally found in vegetables, therefore reducing problematic bloating and gas. For some people it is easy to alternate bites between protein and vegetables, but the main point is that they must be eaten together during each meal to achieve the desired weight loss.

Although it is acceptable to eat protein as a snack by itself, consuming vegetables alone is not encouraged in this program. Eating vegetables alone, without protein to break down the sugar and starch, will cause them to remain in the body longer. To aid in weight loss it is important to eat the two together. **Remember this formula: protein + vegetables = weight loss.**

In this program, we focus on eating 100% natural, unprocessed food with no preservatives. We will only take in foods that are high in protein and low in fat and calories (i.e. turkey, chicken, or fish) with vegetables that are low in carbohydrates but very high in enzymes, vitamins, and minerals (i.e. greens, summer squash, and corn). Corn is higher is carbohydrates but is processed differently by your body. We allow corn every 3 days. Follow the list of appropriate foods.

For your general information, when you eat at least 60-100 grams of protein per day with healthy vegetables, you are consuming about 115 calories from protein per meal and about 60 calories per meal from the vegetables. Compare this to potatoes with condiments such as butter and sour cream, which are 400-600 calories per meal.

You will only consume 600 to 1000 calories per day if you exercise. During the program you will not be counting calories or weighing yourself. As you can see, the low calories you take in are all whole, healthy foods. You will lose inches throughout the body rather than weight. Muscle weighs more than fat, so it will not matter where your weight goes as long as you lose inches and clothing sizes.

When we eat healthy, the lining of our stomachs and intestines becomes clean; therefore, the food is readily absorbed by the body. The cleaner the body, the greater is the amount of absorption. It is important to keep your body clean, particularly during the time of the weight loss. And know that when you eat processed food that includes starch as well as sugar, the starch and sugar remain in your body for three days. If you eat them together, they will remain in the body for six days, and during this period you will not lose weight. It is vital to eat every four hours while in this program; because the body will need to be replenished as whole foods are absorbed quickly. The sugar levels in your body will stabilize as you eat healthy and reduce the fluctuations in your insulin levels. As you eat healthy, your body flushes the toxins and the fat out.

<u>Third Incentive:</u>
Exercise at least three times a week

Exercise is the third most important thing next to eating healthy and preparing your own food. It is very important to add exercise such as walking, aerobics, yoga, or anything else you wish. You may decide to get a personal trainer. By exercising, you are creating lean muscle and therefore building a strong body that burns fat more efficiently.

Make sure to schedule specific times each day when you plan to exercise, in order to create a routine. An hour per day is ideal, but I recommend at least a half an hour a day or one hour, three times a week to achieve greater results with your health and weight loss. People who exercise frequently get double the results compared to people who only eat healthy. This program is different from any other weight loss program you have done because it does not focus solely on losing weight but on being healthy as well as reaching the size you want rather than the weight. Please do not use the scale; instead, measure inches or use clothing sizes and the way your clothes fit.

Fourth Incentive:
Develop a positive sense of self

As you build a strong body by eating healthy and exercising, you must also create a sound mind. The fourth incentive teaches you how to develop a positive sense of self by using affirmations combined with action to create a life that you enjoy, and which will bring you happiness.

Say positive affirmations to yourself throughout the day such as, **"I am strong, I can do this, I am invincible, I have willpower."** When you say these affirmations, it is important not only to believe them with your head, but also in your heart. Believe you can be the person you want to become and tell yourself you can do it each day.

Saying affirmations must be combined with positive actions in order to move you towards your goal. By taking time to reflect on what activity makes you feel alive and gives you energy you will begin to see what steps you can take to make your affirmations a reality. Refer back to Figures 1 and 2 on pages 11-12 about the Cognitive Behavioral Theory we discussed to see how a strong sense of self can be developed.

It is important to cultivate this positive sense of self through reading, meditation, walking, or hobbies that you enjoy so you can find pleasure in doing these things. As you continue to do the above exercise, it will be easy for you to integrate this into your lifestyle. If you visualize a healthy body in the size that you want, you will be able to actualize this on a consistent basis and will be able to maintain your size.

Fifth Incentive:
Create new positive eating habits

Throughout the three sessions as well as while using this book, hypnosis will help to curb and remove your cravings by connecting your mind with your body so you can make the right food choices that will help you achieve your goal. Therefore, you will focus on foods that are healthy for you, as you remove unhealthy ones and develop new, healthy eating habits. Even though your cravings will be eliminated, the habits will still be there. Habits are harder to let go of. They will come back to us when we are in the same circumstances. For example, in the past, in the evenings, I would go for a sweet. The thought will still cross your mind, but it only lasts a few seconds. You will be able to redirect the thought to a new healthy behavior. For example, rather than eating sweets, you will go for a walk, have a cup of tea, read a book, watch a program, etc. Habits are patterns of behavior that we have developed that come back when we do the same action, are in the same environment, or are with the same people. How does this pattern of behavior start? There are times in our life when we feel stressed, have experienced loss, have work or family conflict, any difficulty that a person experiences. The person is reaching out to something to satisfy the emotional desire, something that makes us feel good. This is called emotional hunger. Some people yearn for food, alcohol, shopping, or gambling depending on the unhealthy habit that the person has acquired. We all have bad habits and when we are stressed, they escalate. The first thing you must do is to empty your cupboards of all unhealthy food. If you don't live alone and the others have food that you cannot eat, you may put their food in a different drawer or cupboard, so you do not have access to it.

<u>Sixth Incentive:</u>
Listen to the hypnosis recording daily

The hypnosis recording must be listened to in a sitting position with your back straight, feet on the floor, and hands on your knees so that your body will be grounded, and you will not fall asleep. You will focus on your breathing and visualize a comfortable place where you would like to be. The recording can be listened to anytime when you are alert and can be receptive as well as when you are experiencing difficulties.

The hypnosis recording is a tool to help you to learn to relax. You will visualize your goal and keep it vivid in your mind so you can choose the right foods as well as exercise. Your mind will be able to distinguish between cravings and unhealthy eating habits. As you will see, your cravings will no longer be there. However, your habits may come back during the same time, place, and circumstance but they will only last for a few seconds. You have learned to develop new healthy habits and you will continue to use them. Your positive affirmations will be a great reinforcement throughout the day.

As you remember, our second incentive explains the healthy foods that you need to eat as well as learning how to connect your mind with your body through hypnosis and daily listening of the recording. Through the three sessions as well as the refreshers, the hypnosis is done at the end of each session to facilitate a connection between mind and body. As the visualization about eating healthy becomes clear and strong in your mind, you are eventually able to bring it into your daily life by choosing the right food.

Cravings are removed by the hypnosis. The more you listen to the hypnosis recording, the stronger you reinforce your healthy

29

eating. As you know, we do not consume liquid or products that have caffeine because we believe in natural energy by eating healthy and exercising and getting the appropriate amount of sleep. We use relaxation and hypnosis to connect the mind with the body. This is not only to make the right choices about what a person eats, but also to teach the body how to relax so that this relaxation is repeated throughout the day.

Several hypnosis recordings are included on our website by going to www.thebestyouthroughhypnosis.com. The password to these recordings is "relax".

Just Before You Begin

This book will facilitate your healthy lifestyle program by allowing you to choose what breakfast, lunch, and dinner you prefer. Some ingredients can be exchanged from one recipe to another, and you can adjust according to taste, but always consider the quantity. I have searched through many books, and currently there is nothing written that excludes nuts, fruits, and honey. We eliminate these items on purpose especially during the first few weeks when you need to detoxify your body from sugar, starch, and fat. Know that at the end, most of these foods will be reintroduced.

Additional Information

This program is designed for people ages eighteen and over. Clients outside of this age range can participate in the program, unless otherwise directed by their doctor. For clients under eighteen years of age, fruit, milk, and whole grains are added to the program, because their bodies are still in a growing stage and the foods are necessary. For example, children may have whole wheat toast in the morning as well as ½ cup of fruit per day. It is important to have at least 2-3 servings per day of milk with one serving being plain yogurt with fruit if they wish. If they do not drink milk, they must eat broccoli, shellfish, or orange juice with calcium and vitamin D. We still withhold sweets, sugar, soda, and processed food. Parents must be involved and participate in the food preparation and monitoring.

We offer this program to those who eat meat and fish; however, vegetarians and vegans can also successfully complete the program. We have a special food list for them to follow. This will be given at the first session.

It is important to get at least seven hours of sleep in order for your body to feel healthy and function properly. If you have trouble sleeping, we have a hypnosis recording that can help. In the program, we encourage you to drink at least eight glasses of water per day to cleanse the body as well as to avoid dehydration. We discourage caffeine intake because it may make you agitated and crave the wrong foods, as well as negate the effects of the relaxation. Also, we do not drink any alcohol in the program because the toxins and sugar will not help you to attain your goal. We recommend you prepare your meals in advance so that you can stay on track. The types of recipes in this book are so easy that even a teenager should be able to make them.

It is necessary to take vitamins during the active weight loss portion of this program to avoid hair loss and poor elasticity of your skin. Make sure what you are taking is readily absorbed into your system (powder or liquid form is most effective). A multivitamin as well as 100% of the daily values of Vitamins A, C, E, and a calcium supplement are crucial. You will not get enough A and C because we cut out fruit and E because we cut out grain. Although we know that vegetables do have the above vitamins, people tend to eat a lot of salad and vegetables that are out of season which lack these essential vitamins. For people who need more energy or exercise a lot, you can add B Complex.

The vitamins recommended are available on our website under the "Products for Healthy Living" section.

Stories of Success

We have many success stories. After the three sessions, clients are given a survey to evaluate the program and make suggestions on what to change to increase effectiveness. These are some of their responses:

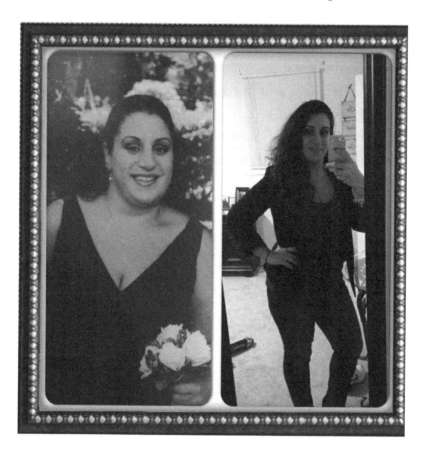

"I learned about the Weight Loss through Hypnosis program through some friends, and I participated in group sessions. When I made my first appointment the description of the program was made clear. I was absolutely given the resources I needed to achieve the goals that I established at the first session. I have reached about 97% of my goal. My start weight in April was 260 lbs (Size 18-20) and I am now 170 lbs (Size 8). - Gina E. (Pictured above)

I learned about Cristina's Weight Loss through Hypnosis program online and participated in the group sessions. The description of the program and expectations were made clear and I feel I was given the resources needed to achieve my goal. Cristina was very supportive and guided me in following this lifestyle program. I have decreased from size 10 to 8 and have lost twelve pounds since starting the program 3 weeks ago. I still have a way to go to reach my goal size of 4 but without the cravings it will be easy to do. It's also a nice feeling to know that free group refreshers are offered if I need them in the future. Cristina is more interested in our success than the money and that says much about her character. I think everything Cristina does to run the program is perfect and I wouldn't change a thing.

-   Pat D.

Absolutely loved the experience and would recommend Cristina to anyone wanting to lose weight. So far, I have lost 55 pounds in 3 months and feel fabulous. It's a great new lifestyle of eating healthy with no cravings! Don't wait...take the first step and give her a call...you won't be disappointed!!

-   Becky B.

I tried almost everything before going to Cristina- all of the diets you hear about, going to the gym, and every time it didn't stick. Now, I've kept it off for over a year, and moreover- I'm so happy. Getting the mind and body aligned is everything- and it wasn't that hard!

-   Liz B.

I have tried Weight loss hypnosis before for a lot more money and in a large impersonal group. Cristina is one-on-one and did an assessment just for me. What a success! Without hesitation I would recommend her to anyone. She really cares about her clients' success and health.

-   Nancy K.

Food List

VEGETABLES
Alfalfa sprouts
Artichokes (any)
Arugula
Asparagus
Avocado (small amount)
Beets/beet greens
Bok Choy
Broccoli
Broccoli rabe
Brussels sprouts
Butternut squash (every 3 days)
Cabbage
Carrots (small amount)
Cauliflower
Celery
Celery root
Collards
Cucumbers
Eggplant
Endive
Fennel
Fiddlehead ferns
Garlic
Kale
Leeks
Mushrooms
Mustard greens
Olives
Onions
Parsnips

Peppers (all kinds)
Pumpkin
Radishes
Romaine lettuce
Rutabaga
Spinach
Spaghetti squash
String beans (yellow or green)
Swiss chard
Tomatoes
Turnips and greens
Watercress
Zucchini
Corn (every 3 days – ½ cup)
Peas (every 3 days – ½ cup)
Lentils (every 3 days – ½ cup)

MILK
Dairy Milk (1%)
Coconut milk
Almond milk
Oat milk
*Dairy milk is to be drunk alone because of the sugar content. Coconut, almond and oat milk should contain no sugar.

Cheeses are allowed, but only fresh and unprocessed. **Only as a condiment, not as a meal.** 100% Milk, no additives, aged is okay.

PROTEIN:

Fish

Anchovies

Bass

Cod

Eel

Flounder

Haddock

Halibut

Herring

Mackerel

Mahi Mahi

Monkfish

Northern pike

Orange roughy

Perch

Red snapper

Rockfish

Salmon

Sardines

Swordfish

Tilapia

Tuna

Walleye

Any other wild fish

SHELLFISH

Abalone

Clams

Crab

Crayfish

Lobster

Mussels

Oysters

Prawns

Scallops

Shrimp

(Fish and shellfish may be eaten every day)

POULTRY

Chicken

Cornish Game Hen

Duck

Emu

Goose

Ostrich

Pheasant

Quail

Turkey

(Poultry may be eaten every day and includes all or any part of the bird)

RED MEAT AND PORK

Beef

Buffalo

Elk

Goat

Lamb

Pork

Rabbit

Venison

(May be eaten 2-3 times per week)

ORGAN MEAT
Liver
Bone marrow
Sweetbreads (brain)
(May be eaten occasionally)

(For your protein: fish, chicken, and turkey have fewer calories than any other meat; therefore, you will lose more weight. Roast, broil, bake, microwave, pan-fry or grill your protein--do not deep-fry it.)

EGGS
Chicken
Duck
Quail
Roe/caviar
Ostrich
(Eggs can be eaten daily. If you have high cholesterol, you may want to omit some or all of the yolk.)

HEALTHY FATS/OILS
(in order of health preference)
Olive oil
Avocado oil
Coconut oil
Grape seed oil
Macadamia oil
Walnut oil
Sesame oil
Lard
Butter/ghee

SPICES AND HERBS
Anise
Basil
Bay Leaf
Black pepper
Cayenne pepper
Chili pepper
Cilantro
Coriander seeds
Cinnamon
Cloves
Cumin
Curcumin
Dill
Fennel
Flax Seeds
Garam Masala
Ginger
Matcha
Mint
Mustard seeds
Nutmeg
Oregano
Paprika
Parsley
Peppermint
Rosemary
Sage
Salt
Stevia leaves
Tarragon
Thyme
Turmeric

OTHER
Aloe Vera
Amla Powder
Apple cider vinegar
Balsamic Vinegar Glaze (very small amount)
Grape Seed Extract (powder)
Vitamins and Supplements
Flax Seeds (every 3 days – ½ cup)
Chia Seeds (every 3 days – ½ cup)
Whole Grain (Farro) (every 3 days – ½ cup)
Matcha
Coffee (1 cup a day) *
Tea (herbal)*
*Creamer or milk is fine. No sugar.

To see which vitamins and nutritional supplements Cristina recommends
https://www.thebestyouthroughhypnosis.com/products
Please consult your doctor if you are taking any medication or are in treatment for an illness.

Scan the QR code to visit Cristina's Product page.

Healthy protein shakes are also allowed to replace one meal. No preservatives, no sugar, stevia leaves okay. Very low in carbohydrates.

FRUIT:
Fresh/frozen Cranberries
Lemons
Limes

Cristina suggests Applegate turkey bacon with no nitrates. However, it is salty so please rinse and pat dry before cooking.

TO BE EXCLUDED:

(Items with an * will be reintroduced to your diet every fourth day after reaching your goal)

Agave*
Alcohol*
Any soda (even diet)
Beans*
Bread*
Brown Rice*
Bulgur wheat*
Cassava*
Cheese, processed
Chickpeas*
Dark chocolate*
Fruit* (except lemon, lime, and fresh cranberries)
Honey (natural)*
Legumes*
Maple syrup (natural)*
Nuts*
Pizza*
Potatoes*
Processed cheeses/American
Quiona*
Rice (white)
Seeds*

Soybeans*
Spaghetti/pasta*
Processed Sugar and Substitutes
Sweet potatoes*
Sweets
Taro*
Wild rice*
Yams*
Yogurt with sugar

Once you have reached your goal, you may consume the starred items in ½ cup portions every fourth day. Cheeses are allowed in small amounts, but only fresh and unprocessed. When reintroducing pasta, bread, or pizza only whole grains will be used. You can reintroduce yogurt without sugar and add fruit to it.

**Please remember to only consume whole, natural, and unprocessed foods. Organic is suggested where available. The food should contain no nitrates, sulfates, preservatives, or MSG

Daily Healthy Lifestyle Program

Week One

Day One

Morning

Glass of water #1* (8 ounces)

*Optional Nutri-Clean cleanse (first week only)

Listen to the hypnosis recording.

Exercise (Make sure you are drinking enough water during exercise)

Glass of water #2 (8 ounces)

The exercise can be done for 30 minutes to one hour. If you are a beginner, start with 15 minutes and then increase it as you go on during the week. You can exercise any time during the day and split up your exercise time if desired. Walk, yoga, aerobics, etc.

Breakfast: Your choice from the menu starting on page 57.

Glass of water #3 15-30 minutes before breakfast

Example: Cristina's Classic Frittata, page 58

Late Morning

Glass of water #4, 15-30 minutes before snack.

Snack (if needed): Your choice from snack recipes starting on page 95.

Example: Romaine and Meat Burrito, page 97

Midday

Glass of water #5, 15-30 minutes before lunch

Lunch: Your choice from lunch recipes starting on page 68.

Example: Simply Chicken Spinach Salad, page 69

Afternoon

Glass of water #6, 15-30 minutes before snack

Snack (if needed): Your choice from snack recipes starting on page 95.

Example: Shrimp Cocktail, page 100

<u>Evening</u>

Glass of water #7, 15-30 minutes before dinner

Dinner: Your choice from dinner recipes starting on page 81.

Example: Turkey Escarole Soup, page 86

Glass of water #8 with dinner.

Evening beverage (optional): if you would also like to have something to drink before bed, you may have tea, seltzer, coconut milk, etc., at least 30 min before bed.

Remember to listen to the hypnosis recording daily to reinforce your healthy lifestyle. Say positive affirmations to yourself daily, throughout the day, to build a positive sense of self. Focus on what is healthy for you and let go of what is unhealthy so you can make the right choices by developing new healthy habits.

<u>Bedtime reflections</u>

Describe here how your day went, how you did with your food and meal plan, any challenges or concerns, triumphs, and anything else you wish to discuss.

_____

_____

_____

_____

<u>Nighttime</u>

Get a good night's sleep of at least 7-8 hours! If you have a hard time sleeping, we do have a hypnosis recording on our website.

In the following space, feel free to describe how your day went, how you did with your food and meal plan, any challenges or concerns, triumphs, and anything else you wish to discuss. Follow the template above.

Day Two:

_____
_____
_____
_____
_____
_____

Day Three:

_____
_____
_____
_____
_____
_____

Day Four:

_____
_____
_____
_____

Day Five:

_____
_____
_____
_____
_____
_____
_____
_____

Day Six:

_____
_____
_____
_____
_____
_____
_____
_____

Day Seven:

_____
_____
_____
_____
_____
_____
_____

End of Week One

Great job! You have now successfully sustained your new healthy lifestyle for a whole week! How do you feel? What did you find to be easier or harder than you first expected? How have you made progress towards your goals this week? Write on these questions in the space below and congratulate yourself on taking care of your body and mind!

_____

_____

_____

_____

_____

_____

_____

_____

_____

_____

_____

_____

_____

_____

_____

_____

_____

_____

Day Eight:

_____

_____

_____

_____

_____

_____

Day Nine:

_____

_____

_____

_____

_____

_____

Day Ten:

_____

_____

_____

_____

_____

_____

_____

Day Eleven:

_____
_____
_____
_____
_____
_____
_____
_____

Day Twelve:

_____
_____
_____
_____
_____
_____

Day Thirteen:

_____
_____
_____
_____
_____
_____

Day Fourteen:

_____

_____

_____

_____

_____

_____

_____

<u>End of Week Two</u>

You are doing wonderfully! Great job tackling that second week! By now you should begin to see the physical results of your new healthy lifestyle. If you feel like the weight isn't coming off as fast as you would like, try to incorporate more exercise in your daily schedule and split some of your meals in half, eating more often and in smaller amounts. Take time to write about your progress this week and where you think you did well and in what ways improvements could be made. Don't forget to pat yourself on the back for all your hard work!

_____

_____

_____

_____

_____

_____

_____

_____

_____

Day Fifteen:

_____

_____

_____

_____

_____

_____

_____

Day Sixteen:

_____

_____

_____

_____

_____

_____

_____

Day Seventeen:

_____

_____

_____

_____

_____

_____

_____

Day Eighteen:

_____

_____

_____

_____

_____

_____

_____

Day Nineteen:

_____

_____

_____

_____

_____

_____

Day Twenty:

_____

_____

_____

_____

_____

_____

Day Twenty-One:

_____
_____
_____
_____
_____
_____
_____

<u>End of Week Three</u>

Congratulations! You've done so well at taking care of your mind and body these past three weeks! Write about the progress you have made in all areas of your life as a result of participating in this program. Give us a call or email and let us know how you did! We love to hear back from you with photos, comments, questions, or concerns.

_____
_____
_____
_____
_____
_____
_____
_____

Week Four and Beyond

You will continue to follow the food plan outlined in the previous three weeks until you reach your goal. As you know, not everybody will reach their goal in just three weeks. It depends on the size you are when you begin the program and the size you want to reach.

It is very important to follow this plan as written, because in the future it is inevitable that you may, at some point, find yourself gaining some weight. This might happen on vacation or over the holidays. The important thing is to continue using the six incentives so that you will still feel good about yourself even with a little weight gain. Remember, one of our goals here is to be confident and happy at any size while working towards a healthy body. So, if you follow the program exactly this time, then when it comes time to lose some weight again you will already have the tools in place to be as successful as you are now.

You will simply go back to eating your lean protein with an equal amount of vegetables, excluding any fruit, starch, or sugar. You will continue to exercise and listen to the hypnosis recording daily. During the first week you may not see any weight loss because the toxins must be flushed out, but by the second week you will see the weight coming off. Continue this until you are again the size at which you feel healthiest.

Imagine You Have Reached Your Goal

You might ask, will I have to eat like this for the rest of my life? Of course not! You must reintegrate healthy food back into your diet, while also maintaining your new healthy lifestyle. The reintroduced foods will include fruit, grains, beans, dairy products, nuts, and certain beverages. But you will continue to avoid heavily processed foods, sodas, artificial sweeteners, and refined sugars because you now understand how harmful those items are to your body.

Maintenance

Now that you have reached your goal you can begin to supplement your healthy diet with the reintroduced foods. Read this part carefully, because I must be very clear about this process, as it is *the most important part* of maintaining your new healthy lifestyle.

In the beginning of the book, we discussed how eating healthy cleans your body of all toxins and leads to a much higher rate of food absorption. This is important to remember, because once you put certain foods back into your body, the traces will remain for several days. Because of this, as we said before, it takes the body three days to flush out the residue from foods such as sugar, starch, carbohydrates, etc. So, every *three to four days* it is okay to include just **one serving** of one of the starred food items in your diet. See page 40 for the list. For example, on Wednesday night you decide to have ½ cup of brown rice with your normal healthy dinner. Now, because you added starch on Wednesday you must wait three days for the body to get rid of the starch before including another food item. Thursday, Friday, and Saturday you eat as you normally would. On Sunday, the fourth day, you can now add one serving (½ cup) of whole-grain pasta to your normal healthy meal that you have for lunch.

As you can see, you will still be eating the way you ate while obtaining weight loss, however these foods will be an *addition* to any one meal in just one serving every three to four days to your diet. It is also important to note that if you for some reason end up having two of these items on any given day it will take your body twice as long to flush out the residue. If you eat both quinoa and a piece of pie on the same day, then you must wait *six* days this time for your body to clean itself.

There are **exceptions** to this rule. Fruit is something that you may enjoy two servings every day. One serving of fruit is one piece or ½ cup of mixed fruit in season. You can eat your fruit at any time of the day including with a snack or any of your three meals. You can also split it up any way you wish. For example, you could decide to have a ½ cup of blueberries one day. You could eat ¼ cup in the morning with breakfast and the other ¼ cup with your afternoon snack.

Nuts and seeds are also okay in small amounts. If you wish to have five or six almonds with your salad at lunch, that is all right. You could also sprinkle some sunflowers seeds on your salad a day or two later. Maybe you would like to have a couple walnuts with your apple another day. Two to three times a week is fine for these.

Honey, agave, or maple syrup are natural sweeteners that can be used sparingly. Perhaps you might like a teaspoon of honey in your coffee or drizzled over your sugar-free yogurt. When used in moderation, these sweeteners can be used a few times a week as well.

The last exception is *only* for people who exercise a lot. By this I mean they work out or do strenuous activity for two to three hours per day several days a week. These people need to have grains included in their diet every day. Just one serving of whole grains will replenish their body of the nutrients that are lost from exercising.

<u>Bottom Line</u>

The bottom line here is that it is your body, and it is up to you to use your best judgment in taking care of it. Not everyone is the same, and you may find that your way of maintaining your healthy lifestyle is a little different from another person's. Maybe you don't like nuts at all, but you find that a couple servings of beans per week give you the energy you need instead.

Remember what you learned here, and you will never have to fear gaining weight or losing control of your eating again. If you make a mistake, don't punish yourself for it. Instead, listen to your body and mind with compassion and love, forgive yourself, and simply wait three more days to clear your body and you will feel healthy again.

With this book, the hypnosis recording, and the six incentives you can't go wrong. You've done great! Now go show the world your new healthy self!

Breakfast Recipes

Cristina's Classic Frittata with Veggies
Servings: 5
Olive oil to coat bottom of pan
10 eggs whites and 3 yolks, beaten
½ cup Cristina's ketchup (page 107)
2 cups Applegate ham or turkey bacon, cooked and cut into pieces.
1½ cups vegetables of choice cooked (asparagus, broccoli, except for kale or spinach ½ cup cooked)
3 stems of parsley leaves, finely chopped
1 tablespoon freshly grated Parmigiano-Reggiano
¼ cup fresh mozzarella or 1 medium mozzarella, cut into pieces
salt and pepper to taste

Preheat oven to 300ºF. In a large bowl, beat the eggs together with the salt and pepper or put in mixer. Set it aside. In a large oven safe non-stick pan over medium heat, add the oil. Pour the egg mixture into the skillet. Drop Cristina's ketchup in and mix around. Sprinkle the Parmigiano-Reggiano and the chopped parsley into the mixture. Add meat and vegetables. Turn off the heat and stir the ingredients to combine. Bake for about 20-25 minutes or until the eggs are set and not runny. Top with pieces of mozzarella and set oven to broil 400°F until mozzarella is melted. Serve directly from the skillet or slice and store for leftovers.
* You can also pour the mixture into muffin cups for individual servings.

Stir-Fry Vegetables with Sliced Turkey Breast
Servings: 1
1 cup assorted veggies, fresh or frozen and cut into 1-inch pieces
½ teaspoon olive oil
4 ounces of cooked turkey breast, cut in ½-inch thick pieces

Heat olive oil in pan on medium heat. Add veggies and sauté until tender to your liking. Add the turkey breast for the last minute, stirring to brown the turkey. Serve warm.

Savory Turkey Bacon and Spinach Egg Muffins
Servings: 2
6 Egg Whites
2 Egg Yolks
8 slices of cooked Applegate turkey bacon
1 cup fresh Spinach, finely chopped
2 tablespoons Parsley, minced
½ cup freshly grated Parmigiano-Reggiano

Preheat oven to 400°F. Blend spinach, parsley, Parmigiano-Reggiano, and eggs together. Dice the turkey bacon and add to egg mixture. Lightly spray a muffin tray with cooking spray. Pour mixture evenly into muffin cups. Bake for 15-20 minutes (check at 15 and then every few minutes, depending on your oven). DON'T OVER COOK. Place leftovers in storage bag and reheat.

Prosciutto, Tomato, and Basil Egg Muffins
Serving Size: 2
6 egg whites
2 egg yolks
8 slices of prosciutto, cut into pieces
½ cup chopped tomatoes (without any liquid)
¼ cup chopped fresh basil
1 tablespoon of freshly grated Parmigiano-Reggiano

Preheat oven to 400°F. Blend tomato, basil, Parmigiano-Reggiano, and eggs together. Add prosciutto to egg mixture. Lightly spray a muffin tray with cooking spray or use muffin liners. Pour mixture evenly into muffin cups. Bake for 15-20 minutes (check at 15 and then every few minutes, depending on your oven). DON'T OVERCOOK. Enjoy 3 muffins and save the rest.

Fried Ham and Turnip Hash
Servings: 1
4 ounces of sliced, all-natural ham
½ cup turnip, peeled and grated
1 scallion, chopped
1 teaspoon olive oil

Wrap grated turnip in paper towels and squeeze out as much liquid as possible. In a small skillet, heat oil over medium heat, add the turnip and scallions, mixing well to coat turnip in the oil. Cook 10-15 minutes, until turnip is nicely browned, stirring occasionally. Fry up your ham in a separate pan or push turnip to the side and fry the ham right in that pan for the last couple minutes. Enjoy.

Southwest Breakfast Scramble
Serving Size: 1
1 teaspoon oil
3 egg whites and 1 egg yolk
4 slices of turkey bacon, cooked and diced
Pinch of sea salt and pepper
5 grape tomatoes, halved
¼ cup minced cilantro or minced parsley
¼ cup small roasted red pepper, diced
¼ avocado, diced

Heat oil in a non-stick skillet over medium heat and sauté all the vegetables. In another non-stick pan over medium heat, cook whisked eggs and add salt and pepper, stirring often. While eggs are still soft, stir in turkey bacon, tomatoes, cilantro or parsley, and red pepper. Top with avocado and serve immediately.

Salmon for Breakfast
Servings: 1
2 teaspoons butter
1 salmon fillet (4-5 ounces)
1 teaspoon dried thyme
½ teaspoon garlic powder
2 teaspoons dried dill
Salt and pepper to taste
1 cup fresh or frozen green beans, trimmed

Preheat oven to 350°F. Grease the bottom of baking dish with half of the butter. Rinse salmon under cool water and pat dry. Place fish flesh side up in baking dish. In a small bowl, melt the remaining butter. Mix your thyme, garlic powder, dill, salt, and pepper to taste. Brush a thin layer over salmon fillet. Bake in the oven for 15-20 minutes or until your salmon is cooked to your liking. Steam the green beans while the salmon cooks, serve together and enjoy!

Breakfast with Espresso Rubbed Steak
Servings: 1
¼ teaspoon chili powder
1 teaspoon finely ground espresso
Kosher salt and pepper to taste
4 ounce serving flank or skirt steak
1 small zucchini

Mix together chili powder, ground espresso, salt, and black pepper. Rub mixture into the steak, covering it completely. Slice steak into thin strips. Heat a little bit of oil in a pan over high heat and add steak, searing for 4-6 minutes or until desired doneness reached. You can also cook on the grill. Slice the zucchini and sauté it with salt and pepper while the steak cooks. Let steak rest and serve.

Shrimp Breakfast Scramble

Servings: 1
½ tablespoon olive oil
¼ yellow onion, minced
3 egg whites
1 egg yolk
4 ounces small, cooked shrimp
½ teaspoon minced fresh dill
½ teaspoon dried basil
2 cooked artichoke hearts, fresh or frozen and defrosted (or a vegetable or your choice)

Heat oil in a small nonstick pan over medium heat. Add onion and sauté until tender, about five minutes. In a medium bowl, beat eggs until frothy. Pour into pan with sautéed onions. Add shrimp, dill, basil, and mix thoroughly until eggs are wet but not completely cooked. Stir in artichoke hearts and finish cooking.

Tuna Topped Spinach Salad

Serving Size: 1
1 cup spinach, or any other leafy green
¼ cup crumbled feta cheese
1 tablespoon dried, unsweetened cranberries, nothing added
3 cherry tomatoes, halved
¼ cup sliced cucumbers
4 ounces tuna, fresh or canned, in oil or water, no additives.
Lemon juice
Olive oil
Salt and pepper to taste

In a bowl mix together spinach, cheese, cranberries, tomatoes, and cucumbers. Top with the tuna. Drizzle lemon juice and olive oil to taste. Add salt and pepper as desired. Enjoy.

One Dish Chicken and Veggies
Serving Size: 2
Olive oil
1 small yellow onion, chopped
1 garlic clove, minced
1 medium carrot, cut into matchsticks
8 ounces fresh asparagus, chopped
10 ounces precooked chicken, cubed
8 ounces fresh, raw spinach
Juice from ½ lemon

In a large skillet, over medium heat, add a drizzle of oil and sauté onion and garlic for about five minutes or until tender. Add asparagus and carrot sticks, continuing to sauté for an additional five minutes. Mix in chicken and stir for one minute. Fold in spinach, remove from heat, and cover. Spinach will wilt from the steam. Remove cover and drizzle mixture with fresh lemon juice.

Turkey Sausage with Peppers and Onions
Serving Size: 1
2 lean chicken or turkey sausage links
1 small red bell pepper, thinly sliced
1 small green or yellow bell pepper, thinly sliced
1 yellow onion, thinly sliced
Olive Oil

Heat one pan with a large drizzle of oil over medium heat. Add peppers and onions and sauté for 8-10 minutes until soft and lightly browned. In a separate pan, sauté sausages over medium heat until fully cooked through. Remove sausage from pan and slice into ¼-inch-thick rounds. Add cut sausage to pan with cooked vegetables and sauté together for an additional 1-2 minutes over medium heat. Season with your choice of herbs and ground black pepper.

Chicken Breakfast Burritos
Serving Size: 1
1 tablespoon olive oil
½ sweet yellow onion, diced
1 garlic clove, pressed
½ red bell pepper, diced
1 teaspoon ground cumin
¼ teaspoon cayenne pepper
4 ounces cooked diced chicken
¼ cup Cristina's sauce (page 109)
½ teaspoon ground black pepper
2 large iceberg or romaine lettuce leaves

Heat olive oil in a large skillet over medium heat. Sauté onion and garlic until tender, about 5 minutes. Toss in bell pepper, cumin, cayenne pepper, and meat, mixing well for one minute. Add sauce and mix with a spatula until cooked thoroughly. Sprinkle with ground pepper. Wrap tightly in lettuce leaves, serve, and enjoy.

Chicken and Kale Salad
Serving Size: 2
1 bunch kale (enough for about 6 cups of chopped leaves)
2 tablespoons olive oil
Juice of 1 small lemon
Sea salt to taste (optional)
¼ teaspoon freshly ground black pepper
2 (4 ounce each) boneless, skinless chicken breasts, cooked

Wash kale and remove leaves from woody stems. Slice leaves thinly. In a large bowl, combine kale, olive oil, lemon juice, sea salt and freshly ground black pepper. Toss half of kale to coat leaves completely and transfer to a medium bowl. Top the salad with one chicken breast, sliced. Cover and save the rest of the dressing, kale, and chicken for tomorrow.

Chili-Lime Shrimp Sauté with Cherry Tomatoes
Servings: 1
1 tablespoon olive oil
½ clove garlic, minced
¼ cup cherry tomatoes, sliced in half
4 ounces medium shrimp
½ teaspoon paprika
1 tablespoon parsley or cilantro, chopped
Half a lime for juice
Cayenne pepper, to taste

Heat oil in a skillet over medium heat. Add garlic and sauté for 1 minute. Add tomatoes and cook for 2 minutes, stirring. Toss in shrimp and cook for an additional 2-3 minutes. Shrimp is done when pink. Turn off heat and toss with paprika and parsley cilantro. Squeeze lime juice over shrimp and sprinkle on cayenne pepper to taste.

Quick and Easy Chicken Sausage Veggie Sauté
Servings: 1
1 chicken sausage, chopped and semi-cooked
¼ small onion, chopped
1 medium zucchini, spiral sliced or chopped and dried
3 fresh mushrooms, chopped
1 tablespoon olive oil
Salt and pepper to taste

Drizzle oil in a large skillet and heat over medium-high heat. Add in onion and chicken sausage. Sauté until lightly browned, 2-3 minutes. Add zucchini and mushroom and toss to mix with onion and sausage. Sprinkle with salt and pepper to taste and cook for 2 minutes, until veggies are as tender as you like them.

Spaghetti Squash Omelet

Servings: 2
1 cup spaghetti squash, cooked (Page 110)
3 egg whites
1 egg yolk
¼ cup freshly grated Parmigiano-Reggiano
1 tablespoon of olive oil
Salt and pepper to taste
6 slices turkey bacon, cooked, and chopped

Whisk eggs, then mix them with the squash and add salt and pepper to taste. In a 10-inch pan, over medium heat, warm the olive oil. Add the egg mixture to the pan and spread it out evenly. Let it cook for 1 minute and add the turkey bacon. Put a lid on the pan and cook for 1-2 minutes more. Use a spatula to gently fold the omelet in half, and then slide it out of the pan. Cut in half and use the remaining serving for the next day.

Baked Stuffed Tomato & Egg Breakfast with Turkey Bacon

Serving Size: 1
2 medium/large fresh tomatoes
2 large eggs
1 teaspoon fresh Italian parsley
1 slice turkey bacon, cooked and chopped
Sea salt & cracked black pepper to taste

Preheat oven to 350°F. Line a baking sheet with aluminum foil. Cut the tops of the tomatoes off. With a spoon, scoop out all the tomato innards. Crack an egg in each hollowed-out tomato. Bake for 30 minutes. Let cool for a few minutes. Top with crumbled turkey bacon. Dust with minced parsley, salt & pepper and enjoy!

Prosciutto and Spinach Poached Eggs
Serving Size: 1
2 Roma tomatoes, halved lengthways
½ tablespoon olive oil
Salt and pepper to taste
½ tablespoon basil leaves, chopped
4 slices prosciutto
1 cup water
Splash white wine vinegar
2 eggs
½ cup baby spinach

Preheat oven to 350°F. Place tomatoes on a baking tray, and drizzle with oil, basil, salt, and pepper to taste. Arrange prosciutto on a baking tray lined with parchment paper. Bake tomatoes for 10-15 minutes, or until they begin to collapse. Place the tray with prosciutto in the oven for the last 5 minutes. Meanwhile, poach eggs by cracking them gently into a frying pan of slightly simmering water with a splash of vinegar (helping the eggs to set). Continue simmering, occasionally splashing hot water over eggs, for 2-3 minutes or until desired temperature is reached. Serve tomatoes and prosciutto with poached eggs on top, over a bed of baby spinach.

Lunch Recipes

Simply Chicken Spinach Salad
Servings: 2
2 cups spinach
3 olives
¼ cup sliced cucumber
¼ cup broccoli florets
¼ cup sliced bell peppers, any color you like
12 ounces cooked chicken breast or other protein, cut into pieces
Lemon juice
Olive oil
Salt and pepper

Combine veggies and protein in a large bowl. Add lemon and salt and pepper. Stir well, then seal the flavor with olive oil and enjoy.

Beef and Butternut Squash Stew
Servings: 4
2 tablespoon olive oil
1 small onion, cut into pieces
2 cloves garlic, whole
1 tablespoon fresh rosemary, minced
1 tablespoon fresh thyme, chopped
2 pounds beef stew meat, cut into 2-inch cubes
1 lb. butternut squash, cut into 2-inch cubes
¼ cup sun dried tomatoes
4 tablespoons tomato paste, no preservatives
3 cups Cristina's broth (page 106)

In a large soup pot, heat olive oil on medium heat. Add onions, garlic, rosemary, thyme, and sauté until onions are tender. Turn up heat, add beef and cook until meat is browned. Add sun dried tomatoes and tomato paste. Stir to combine. Next add broth. Be sure to add enough broth so that beef and squash are completely covered and stir to combine. Bring to a boil over high heat then reduce to a simmer. Cover and allow to cook for 1 hour or more. In the last ½ hour add the squash. Add salt and pepper to taste. If you want the squash to be softer, continue to cook until you have the right texture.

Cristina's Turkey Burgers with Grated Zucchini and Carrots

Servings: 4

1 cup Cristina's Ketchup (page 107)
1-pound lean ground turkey
1 zucchini, grated
1 carrot, grated
1 full egg
Handful of parsley, finely minced
1 tablespoon grated Parmigiano-Reggiano
Salt, pepper, and spices to taste
Lettuce, tomato, and onion as desired

In a pot, over medium heat, cook grated carrot for one minute in the ketchup and remove from heat. Add grated zucchini. Break an egg and mix together all ingredients, remembering to season well. Using hands, squish everything together until all is well combined. Form into patties. Preheat a nonstick pan to medium heat. Cook for a few minutes on each side. Serve with lettuce, tomato, onion, or other desired veggies. Enjoy the burgers as a snack or a full meal with your whole family. Save additional burgers for the next day.

Italian Sausage Mushroom Caps

Serving Size: 2

12 small, bite size mushroom caps, stems removed
¾-pound Italian sausage, casing removed
¼ cup feta cheese or goat cheese, crumbled

Preheat oven to 350°F. Shape the sausage into 12 meatballs. Place the meatballs into the mushroom caps. Using the tip of a knife create a hole in the top of each meatball. Place a small goat cheese or feta crumble into each hole. Place mushrooms on a baking sheet and put them into the oven for 15-20 minutes or until meat has cooked through. Enjoy.

Endive Salmon Poppers

Servings: 1
1 head endive
4 ounces smoked salmon
½ red onion, minced
¼ avocado, sliced
Salt and pepper to taste
1 tablespoon olive oil

Separate endive leaves. Top with smoked salmon, red onion, and avocado. Sprinkle with salt and pepper to taste. Drizzle olive oil over the top and serve.

Peppercorn Tuna Skewers with Eggplant

Servings: 2
1 tablespoon or less of multicolored peppercorns
1 teaspoon paprika
2- 6oz servings good quality fresh tuna, cubed
1 large eggplant, cut into ¼ inch thick pieces
1 tablespoon of your favorite vinegar
1 clove garlic, minced
1 tablespoon basil, chopped
2 tablespoons of olive oil

Heat your grill to high heat. Soak short wooden skewers in water for about 30 minutes. In a spice grinder, grind the peppercorns finely. In a bowl combine the ground pepper, salt and the paprika. In another bowl whisk together vinegar, garlic, basil, and olive oil. Add the tuna cubes to the first bowl and toss to coat. Swirl the eggplant slices in the second bowl to evenly coat. Place eggplant on the grill, close the lid and turn after about 3-5 minutes. Cook another few minutes then remove. Drizzle eggplant with olive oil and season to taste. Thread the tuna cubes on skewers, and drizzle with a little more olive oil. Grill the skewers, turning brown on all sides, until seared on the outside and still pink in the center 2-4 minutes. You may use the other serving for another day.

Tasty Chicken Cutlet Sandwich

Servings: 2
8-ounce chicken breast, pounded flat to make a cutlet
1 teaspoon freshly grated Parmigiano-Reggiano
4 slices ¾" thick eggplant
¼ cup avocado
1 lemon wedge
Tomato and lettuce as desired

Preheat oven to 350°F. Grill the chicken cutlet and eggplant on the grill for about five minutes. The chicken should be just about cooked through, and the eggplant will have browned nicely. Transfer chicken and eggplant to a baking sheet and sprinkle the Parmigiano-Reggiano onto the chicken. Pop into preheated oven for 3-5 minutes until cheese has melted and eggplant is still firm but moist. Combine avocado and juice from the lemon wedge, add salt and pepper if desired. Spread avocado mixture onto one piece of the eggplant "bread," add chicken, top with lettuce and tomato, put the other slice of eggplant on top and enjoy your sandwich.

Spaghetti Squash with Pesto

Servings: 2
8-ounce roasted chicken, cut into small pieces
2 cups cooked spaghetti squash (page 110)
1 cup pesto with no nuts (page 109)
1 cup cherry tomato, quartered
Basil to garnish (optional)

Toss the squash with the chicken, tomatoes, and pesto in a pot over medium heat until well combined and warmed. Garnish with fresh basil if desired.

Delightful Salmon with Garlic, Spinach, and Tomatoes

Servings: 4

4 skinless salmon fillets (6 ounces each), rinsed and patted dry
2 cups fresh spinach
¼ cup shallots, minced
4 garlic cloves, minced
5 sun-dried tomatoes, chopped
¼ teaspoon red pepper flakes
Sea salt and freshly ground black pepper to taste
1 tablespoon olive oil

Preheat oven to 350°F. Season each salmon filet with salt and pepper to taste and line up in a baking dish. Place it in the oven. Bake for 10 to 15 minutes or until the fish is just cooked through. Heat oil in a skillet over medium heat. Add shallots and cook until soft, about 3 minutes, stirring occasionally. Add garlic and cook for another minute. Add spinach, sun-dried tomatoes, and pepper flakes. Cook for another 2 to 3 minutes and season to taste. Remove vegetables from heat and serve with salmon.

Red Snapper Scampi with Steamed Veggies

Servings: 2

1 tablespoon butter, melted
Splash white wine
1 clove garlic finely minced
Lemon peel to grate
Salt and pepper to taste
½-pound red snapper
2 cups mixed veggies of choice, chopped

Preheat oven to 450°F. Combine melted butter, wine, garlic, lemon peel, and pepper in a small bowl and stir to blend. Place the fish in a parchment lined baking pan. Top with the seasoned butter. Bake 8 to 10 minutes or until the fish begins to flake easily with a fork. While the fish cooks, steam your veggies over the stove until as tender as you like. Salt and pepper to taste and top with scampi.

Lamb with Sweet Red Peppers
Servings: 2
½-pound boneless leg of lamb, cut into 1" pieces
Sea salt and pepper to taste
1 tablespoon olive oil
1 garlic clove, minced
1 cup Cristina's broth, hot (page 106)
2 large red bell peppers, sliced into rings
1 tablespoon fresh parsley, chopped

Rub lamb with sea salt and freshly ground black pepper. Set it aside.
Heat a large skillet over high heat and add olive oil when hot. Brown
the lamb on all sides, turning frequently (3-5 minutes). Add garlic and
broth to the pan with the lamb and bring to a boil. Once boiling,
reduce heat to medium, and cook partially covered for 30 minutes.
Uncover and cook 10-15 minutes longer, or until the lamb is tender
enough to fall apart with a fork. Add red peppers and cook for
another 10 minutes, or until peppers are tender. Top with fresh
parsley.

Healthy Pizza with Homemade Cauliflower Crust
Servings: 4
4 cups raw cauliflower rice (1 medium sized head of cauliflower)
1 egg, beaten
1/3 cup of fresh Parmigiano-Reggiano
1 teaspoon dried oregano
Pinch of salt
1-2 cups Cristina's Ketchup (page 107) or your favorite salsa
½ lb. of Prosciutto, bacon, or another meat
1 cup of fresh mozzarella cheese

Preheat oven to 400°F. To make cauliflower rice, pulse batches of raw
cauliflower florets in a food processor until a rice-like texture is
achieved. Steam cauliflower rice until tender or cook in microwave
until tender. In a large bowl, mix cooked cauliflower rice, beaten egg,
Parmigiano-Reggiano, and spices. It needs to be mixed very well so

74

don't be afraid to use your hands. It won't be like any pizza dough you've ever worked with, but it will hold together as you cook it. Press dough onto a baking sheet lined with parchment paper. Keep dough about 1/3-inch thick and make edges slightly higher for crust. Bake for 35-40 minutes. The crust should be golden brown and firm when finished. Add sauce, cheese, and meat as desired and return pizza to the oven. Cook an additional 5-10 minutes, just until the cheese is hot and bubbly. Enjoy it and share with family.

Crock Pot Pork Loin
Servings: 5
1 boneless pork loin (about 3 pounds)
2 cups Cristina's ketchup (page 107)
2 small zucchini, diced
2 Celery stalks, cut into small pieces
2 Carrots, cut into pieces
2 small head cauliflower, separated into florets
1 teaspoon basil, chopped
2 cup red wine
1 cup Cristina's broth (page 106)
Salt and pepper to taste

Marinate overnight with 1 cup of wine, salt, pepper, and any spices you like. Preheat crock-pot to high. Light your grill and turn to high. When it is ready, brown the pork loin until it is crusty on the outside but red on the inside. Keep turning the pork loin as you go. You can lower the heat, so it does not burn. If you don't have a grill, you can use a nonstick pot with a drizzle of olive oil and brown as if you were using the grill. Turn continually until browned. Take loin and place in the hot crock pot with ketchup, basil, carrots, and celery. Add one glass of wine and 1 cup of Cristina's broth. Let cook for two hours. When meat is almost cooked, in the last ½ hour, add zucchini and cauliflower. You could also simmer in a stock pot over the stove on low for about the same amount of time, depending on your stove.

Mediterranean-Style Tuna with Garlic, Parsley, and Tomatoes

Servings: 2
2 Yellowfin tuna steaks (4-5 ounce each)
¼ teaspoon salt
¼ teaspoon ground coriander
Pinch black pepper
Cooking spray
6-7 cherry tomatoes
1 tablespoon green onion, chopped
2 teaspoons parsley
½ tablespoon capers, drained
½ tablespoon olive oil
½ tablespoon lemon juice
¼ teaspoon minced garlic
6 pitted Kalamata olives, chopped

Heat a large nonstick skillet over medium-high heat. Sprinkle fish with half of the salt, coriander, and pepper. Coat pan with cooking spray. Add fish to pan, cook 4 minutes on each side or until desired degree of doneness. While fish cooks, combine remaining salt, spices, tomato, and remaining ingredients. Serve tomato mixture over fish. You may choose to sauté all of your vegetables and serve over your fish.

Rustic Breadless Chicken with Artichokes

Servings: 2
2 cups skinless, boneless chicken breast, diced and cooked
2 cups artichoke hearts, fresh or frozen
3 large tomatoes, cut into small wedges
¼ cup black olives, halved
¼ cup fresh basil, chopped
2 tablespoons olive oil
2 tablespoons white wine vinegar
1 tablespoon freshly pressed lemon juice
Sea salt and black pepper, to taste

Heat pans with a drizzle of olive oil and a tablespoon of water over low heat. Add artichoke hearts and season to taste. Cook artichokes until tender. Transfer to a large salad bowl. Add chicken, tomatoes, olives, and fresh basil to the bowl, and toss to combine. In a small bowl, combine ingredients for the vinaigrette with remaining oil. Season to taste and mix well. Drizzle vinaigrette over the salad, toss, and serve.

Traditional Italian Fish Stew

Servings: 2
2 skinless cod or sea bass fillets, 4 ounces each
1 cup shrimp, peeled and deveined
1/3 cup onion, chopped
2 stalks celery, sliced
1 clove garlic, minced
2 teaspoons olive oil
1 cup Cristina's broth (page 106)
¼ cup dry white wine, if desired (or substitute with broth)
1 ¾ cup of diced tomatoes
1 cup Cristina's sauce (page 109)
1 teaspoon oregano
¼ teaspoon salt
1/8 teaspoon ground black pepper
1 tablespoon fresh parsley, minced

Rinse fish and shrimp, pat dry with paper towels. Cut fish into 1 ½-inch pieces. Cut shrimp in half lengthwise. Cover and chill fish and shrimp until needed. In a large saucepan or stockpot, cook onion, celery, and garlic in oil until tender. Stir in Cristina's broth and white wine. Bring to a boil and stir, reduce heat to simmer, uncovered, for five minutes. Stir in fish next, return to just boiling. Reduce heat to low. Cover and simmer for three to five minutes, or until fish flakes easily with a fork and shrimp are opaque. Enjoy half and save the other portion for later.

Baked Italian-Style Portabella Mushrooms with Prosciutto and Mozzarella

Servings: 2
4 large portabella mushroom caps
4 cloves garlic, minced
¾ cup Cristina's Sauce (page 109)
½ red bell pepper, chopped
¼ medium yellow onion, chopped
4 ounces fresh mozzarella cheese, diced
8 slices prosciutto, chopped
Italian seasoning (if desired)
Olive oil
Salt and pepper, to taste

Heat oven to 350°F. Clean the mushrooms with wet paper towels, remove stems and set aside. Place mushroom caps upside down on a pan and drizzle with olive oil and minced garlic. Salt lightly. Place mushrooms in oven for 10 minutes while preparing filling. Chop mushroom stems into medium pieces and combine with Cristina's Sauce, pepper, and onion in a medium bowl. Remove mushroom caps from oven and fill with sauce mixture. Top mushroom with prosciutto and cheese. Sprinkle several shakes of Italian seasoning over the top of each cap (if desired). Place in oven for 10 minutes, until mixture is heated through, and cheese is melted and starting to brown. Remove from oven and serve immediately.

Turkey and Veggie Fajitas

Servings: 3
1 tablespoon olive oil
1 small garlic clove, crushed
½ lime for juice
¼ teaspoon chili powder
¼ teaspoon ground cumin
¾ pound turkey cutlets, cut into ½ inch strips
½ small yellow onion, cut into 8 wedges
½ red bell pepper, cut into ½ inch strips

½ yellow bell pepper, cut into ½ inch strips
1/8 cup parsley, chopped
½ small bunch scallions, thinly sliced
½ cup Cristina's ketchup (page 107)
¼ cup sour cream, optional

Combine oil with garlic, lime juice, chili powder, and cumin in a large bowl. Add turkey and mix well. Cover and refrigerate for at least two hours. Remove from refrigerator thirty minutes prior to cooking. Heat the remaining 2 teaspoons of olive oil in skillet over medium heat. Add onion and peppers and cook for 10 minutes, stirring occasionally. Toss in turkey and cook for additional 10 minutes, stirring continuously. Scatter in parsley and sliced scallions. Serve topped with Cristina's ketchup, and sour cream if desired.

Cristina's Minestrone Soup

1 medium onion, diced
4 carrots, diced
4 stalks of celery, diced
2 cups zucchini, diced
2 cups cabbage, blanched and cut in small pieces
five tomatoes, peeled, diced
2 cups butternut squash, diced
1 cup peas
2 cups string beans, chopped
2 cloves of garlic, minced
4 cups Cristina's Chicken and Beef Broth (page 106)
Salt and Pepper to taste
2 tablespoons Olive Oil

Add olive oil to a heavy bottom pot and turn the heat on to medium-high. Add the onion and cook for 3-4 minutes or until the onion is soft and translucent. Add garlic and tomatoes. Cook tomatoes until soft and blended with onion. Make sure to add salt and pepper. Add remaining vegetables. Cook until tender and a little crunchy. You may add ½ cup of white wine to deglaze the bottom of the pan. Add broth, salt and pepper and simmer until vegetables are cooked to the consistency that you prefer. This recipe can be frozen. Feel free to make small meatballs or add chicken to this if desired.

Dinner Recipes

Cristina's Stuffed Turkey Eggplant Rollatini

Servings: 6
1 ½ pound ground turkey
½ pound ground pork
4 medium eggplants
4 cups of Cristina's sauce (page 109)
1 medium fresh mozzarella (chopped into small pieces)
½ cup freshly grated Parmigiano-Reggiano
½ cup parsley, fresh, minced
3 eggs
½ pound whole milk ricotta cheese
1 teaspoon nutmeg
Olive oil
Salt and pepper to taste along with any spices to taste

Preheat oven to 375°F. Season the meat with salt and pepper and sauté. Break the meat apart as you cook. If you need to break it apart more, put it in the blender and pulse a few times until fine. Set aside and let cool. Mix ricotta and nutmeg. When the meat is cool, mix the meat, ricotta mixture, eggs, parsley, mozzarella, Parmigiano-Reggiano, and salt and pepper to make the filling. Skin the eggplant. Cut off both ends and cut lengthwise into 1/8-inch slices. Grill on both sides until they are cooked but still flexible. Salt the eggplant. Brush one side with olive oil and spoon as much filling as you would like onto the eggplant. Put a small amount of sauce over the filling. Roll and place in baking dish in a single layer. If using foil baking dish, please double so it will not burn. Spoon the remaining sauce over roll-ups. Sprinkle with some Parmigiano-Reggiano cheese. Cover and bake for 15-20 minutes. Uncover and bake an additional 15 minutes or until bubbly. Enjoy with your whole family.

Classic Chicken Parmesan

Servings: 2
8 ounces chicken breast, in 2 pieces
2 tablespoons of olive oil
2 thin slices of fresh mozzarella cheese
4 basil leaves + 1 tablespoon fresh chopped basil
½ cup of freshly grated Parmigiano-Reggiano
½ cup Cristina's Sauce (page 109)
1 ½ cups spiralized* or julienned vegetables of your choice (We chose
parsnips, zucchini, and yellow squash)
½ lemon for juice

Preheat oven to 350°F. In blender, add Parmigiano-Reggiano and 1 tablespoon of basil and blend in pulsating motion. Coat chicken breast in half of the olive oil. Roll chicken in Parmigiano-Reggiano and basil mixture. Bake for 15 minutes in your preheated oven. Remove chicken from oven and top with mozzarella and Cristina's Sauce. Put chicken back in the oven and bake for a few more minutes until the mozzarella is melted. Heat a splash of olive oil in a large pan over medium-high heat. When the pan is hot, stir fry your vegetables for a minute or two, until tender. Remove veggies from heat and top with lemon juice, the rest of the basil, and salt and pepper to taste. Serve the chicken over vegetables and enjoy. You could also serve it over a freshly made salad if you prefer.

*To spiralize the vegetables you can choose from a few different methods. A spiralizer is a device you can buy from any home goods store nearby. If you don't have one or want to get one a julienne blade attached to your regular vegetable peeler works almost as well. And an alternative to that method would be to simply grate or slice the vegetables thinly.

Slow-Cooked Spanish Cod

Servings: 2
Pinch of saffron threads
3 tablespoons dry white wine (no preservatives or sulfates)
1 tablespoon olive oil
2 cloves of garlic peeled, but left whole
1 bay leaf
1 plum tomato, seeded and coarsely chopped
¼ cup vegetable stock, all natural
Salt and pepper
2 cod fillets (4 ounces each)
1 small red bell pepper, seeded and finely chopped
2 teaspoons coarsely chopped fresh parsley
1 teaspoon sherry vinegar

Soak the saffron in 1 tablespoon of white wine for 20 minutes. In a large frying pan warm ½ tablespoon of olive oil over low heat. Add the garlic cloves and cook lightly, stirring occasionally until tender but not browned, about 10 minutes. Add the remaining 2 tablespoons of wine and transfer the contents of pan to a slow cooker. Stir in the bay leaf, tomatoes, the saffron mixture, the stock, and salt to taste. Cover and cook on low for about 2 hours. Stir and add the Cod, cover, and continue cooking for 15 more minutes, until the fish flakes easily with a fork. Add the diced bell pepper, parsley, vinegar and the remaining ½ tablespoon of oil. Season with salt and pepper and stir gently to combine. Serve half and save the rest for lunch tomorrow.

Scallops and Asparagus Entree

Servings: 1
5 medium scallops
2 teaspoons olive oil
1 tablespoon yellow onion, minced
1 teaspoon parsley, chopped

Lemon wedge, for garnish
6 stalks asparagus, trimmed

Heat olive oil in a large skillet over medium heat. Add asparagus to a small sauté pan with ½ inch of water, heat over medium-low, and cover pan. When skillet is hot, add in onion. Sauté, stirring frequently for 1 to 2 minutes, or until lightly browned. Add scallops and cook for 1 minute on each side until brown. Check asparagus; remove from heat when tender to your liking. Take scallops and onion out of pan immediately once opaque and season with salt and pepper to taste. Top with parsley and serve with lemon wedge and steamed asparagus.

Tangy Salsa Chicken
Servings: 4
2 tablespoons minced fresh parsley or cilantro
3 tablespoons fresh lime juice
1 ½ tablespoons olive oil
4 (4 ounce) skinless, boneless chicken breast halves
½ teaspoon salt
Cooking spray
1 cup chopped plum tomato
2 tablespoons chopped onion
Pepper to taste
¼ avocado, peeled and finely chopped

To prepare chicken, combine parsley or cilantro, 2 ½ tablespoons of the lime juice, olive oil, and the chicken breasts in a large bowl. Toss ingredients and let settle for 3 minutes. Remove the chicken from marinade and discard the rest. Sprinkle chicken evenly with ¼ teaspoon of salt. Heat your grill and coat the surface of it with cooking spray. Add chicken to the grill and cook for 6 minutes on each side or until done. (If you don't have a grill you can bake in the oven at 350 for 10–15 minutes, or sauté over medium-high heat

3-4 minutes each side). The chicken is done when the inside is no longer pink, and the juices run clear. To prepare salsa, combine tomato, remaining lime juice, onion, and pepper in a medium bowl. Add avocado; stir gently to combine. Serve salsa over the chicken. Enjoy with the rest of your family or refrigerate/freeze the leftovers.

Turkey Escarole Soup
Servings: 3
2 cups stewed tomatoes, chopped
2 cups Cristina's broth (page 106)
1 pound cooked diced or shredded turkey
2 cups roughly chopped escarole (1 medium head)

Combine the tomatoes and broth in a small stockpot. Bring to a boil, then reduce heat to low, cover and simmer for 5 minutes. Add the turkey, escarole stirring to combine. Cook for an additional 5 minutes over low. Serve and enjoy.

Stuffed Peppers with Ground Chicken
Servings: 2
3 large, sweet bell peppers, any color
4-ounce can, diced green chilies, no preservatives
½ pound ground chicken
1 tablespoon parsley, chopped
¼ cup onion, chopped
1 teaspoon cumin
½ teaspoon chili powder
½ teaspoon salt
1 cup of Cristina's sauce (page 109)
1 tablespoon of Parmigiano-Reggiano

Preheat oven to 350°F. In a medium sized bowl mix diced chilies with chicken, parsley, onion, cumin, chili powder and salt. Cut the tops off of the sweet peppers and set aside. Remove seeds and the white part. Place peppers in a baking dish. Stuff peppers with the

chicken mixture; sprinkle with Parmigiano-Reggiano and cover
with sauce. Cover and bake for 1 hour. Enjoy and save any
leftovers.

Scrumptious Spanish Spaghetti Squash with Olives
Servings: 2
1 pound spaghetti squash, cooked
1 tablespoon olive oil
1 cup chopped onion
2 teaspoons minced garlic
1 teaspoon dried oregano
½ teaspoon celery salt
¼ teaspoon crushed red pepper
¼ teaspoon freshly ground black pepper
¼ teaspoon crushed saffron threads, optional
1-pound extra-lean ground beef
1 2/3 cups Cristina's sauce (page 109)
2 ounces (about ½ cup) pimiento-stuffed olives, sliced
¼ cup dry sherry
1 tablespoon capers
¼ cup chopped fresh parsley, divided
1-2 tablespoons of Parmigiano-Reggiano

Heat a large skillet over medium-high heat, adding oil to pan, swirl
to coat. Add onion and sauté for 4 minutes or until tender. Add
garlic, sauté for 1 minute. Next, stir in oregano, celery salt, red
pepper, black pepper and saffron if desired. Add ground beef; cook
5 minutes or until beef is browned, stirring to crumble. Stir in
Cristina's sauce, olives, dry sherry, capers and 3 tablespoons of
parsley. Bring to a boil. Reduce heat and simmer for 15 minutes.
Add spaghetti squash to mixture. Cook for 2 minutes or until
thoroughly heated. Sprinkle with remaining parsley and
Parmigiano-Reggiano and enjoy!

Grilled Chicken with Lemon and Rosemary

Servings: 2
1-pound skinless, boneless chicken breast
2 tablespoons olive oil
¼ cup lemon juice
2 cloves garlic, pressed
¼ cup fresh rosemary, minced
½ teaspoon sea salt

In a medium bowl, combine olive oil, lemon juice, garlic, rosemary, and salt. Rinse chicken breasts, pat dry and place in a 7 x 11-inch baking dish. Pour marinade over chicken, cover, and refrigerate for at least 30 minutes or up to 6 hours. Heat grill and cook chicken for 5-7 minutes per side until browned and cooked in the center. Serve with vegetable of choice.

Spaghetti with Meatballs

Servings: 4
1 tablespoon olive oil
3 cups Cristina's sauce (page 109)
20 Cristina's Meatballs, medium (page 108)
24 ounces kelp noodles (or one spaghetti squash)

Heat a large skillet over medium-high heat. Add sauce and meatballs and bring to a simmer. Serve over spaghetti squash or prepared kelp noodles. Add to the skillet with the meatballs and sauce. Save the rest for the next day.

Healthy Shepherd's Pie

Servings: 2
½ pound ground beef, turkey, or chicken
1 clove garlic, minced
¼ medium yellow onion, chopped
½ large carrot, chopped
½ cup fresh or frozen peas or corn
1 teaspoon fresh rosemary, chopped
½ teaspoon fresh thyme
½ cup Cristina's Broth (Page 106) or beef consommé
2 teaspoons Worcestershire Sauce
½ small butternut squash, washed and dried
1 tablespoon coconut milk or butter
Small pat of butter
Sea salt and pepper, to taste
Cooking spray

Preheat oven to 325°F. In a medium skillet, brown meat and break apart over medium-high heat. Once meat is browned, drain grease from pan and set meat aside. Cook onions and carrots in a drizzle of olive oil until carrots are soft and onions translucent. Add meat back to pan, add broth or beef consommé, rosemary, thyme, and salt. Continue to cook at medium-low heat until all excess liquid has cooked off. Stir in peas or corn. Pour meat mixture into a small baking dish that has been coated with cooking spray. Pierce the butternut squash all over with a sharp knife while the meat is cooking. Place in shallow dish and microwave on high for about 5-8 minutes, depending on microwave strength. Remove squash, cut in half, and scoop out pulp and seeds with a spoon. Scoop cooked squash and place into a medium-sized bowl with coconut milk, butter, sea salt and pepper. Mash into a paste and spread on top of meat mixture. Bake for 10 to 15 minutes, or until the sides are bubbling and the center is hot. Enjoy a serving for dinner tonight and save the rest for tomorrow.

*You can also substitute butternut squash for mashed cauliflower.

Chicken Nuggets with Carrot

Servings: 2
8 ounces ground chicken
1 tablespoon parsley, chopped
1 scallion, chopped
1 egg
2 tablespoons olive oil
½ cup coconut flour
Pinch of nutmeg
Salt and pepper, to taste
¼ cup Cristina's Ketchup (page 107)
2 large carrots, diced into ¾-inch sticks
Coarse salt, to taste

Mix together the chicken, parsley, scallion, and the egg. Heat a small skillet over medium and add the olive oil, swirling to evenly coat the pan. Put coconut flour on a small plate or in a shallow bowl. Make 4-5 small nuggets out of the chicken mixture with your hands and coat them very lightly in the coconut flour. Place nuggets in the skillet an inch apart and cook for 4 minutes, turn, and keep them in for another 4 minutes. Chicken nuggets are done when both sides are golden and crispy, and the chicken is cooked through. For the carrot fries, reheat oven to 425°F. Toss carrot sticks in a bowl with the rest of the olive oil to coat. Place the sticks on a parchment paper lined baking sheet and sprinkle with coarse salt. Bake for 15 minutes, flip and cook for 10 more minutes. Serve the carrot and nuggets with Cristina's Ketchup and enjoy!

Eggplant Lasagna

Servings: 4-6
2 tablespoons olive oil, divided
3 medium-sized eggplants, sliced lengthwise
1 ½ lb. ground mild Italian sausage meat
2 shallots, diced
2 garlic cloves, minced
1 tablespoon fresh basil, minced
1 teaspoon dried oregano
Salt and pepper to your liking
4 cups Cristina's sauce (page 109)
½ lb. 100% whole milk ricotta
2 large mozzarella (12oz) or 3 medium mozzarella (8oz), cut into small pieces
3 tablespoon plus 1 tablespoon freshly grated Parmigiano-Reggiano

Preheat oven to 400°F. With one tablespoon of olive oil, lightly brush each side of your sliced eggplant. Roast the eggplant slices on a baking sheet for 10 minutes. Meanwhile, heat another tablespoon of olive oil over medium heat. Add the Italian sausage along with half of the shallots and garlic. Continue to cook until sausage is browned. Remove from heat and set aside. By this time, the eggplant slices should be done. Remove from the oven and set aside to cool slightly. While the oven is still hot, spoon a small amount of Cristina's sauce onto the bottom of a 9" ×13" baking dish. This will prevent the bottom layer of eggplant from sticking. Next, layer your ingredients — the eggplant, the sausage, sauce, and the three cheeses. Repeat making three layers— until all ingredients are used up. Sprinkle the top of your dish with the Parmigiano-Reggiano and cover with sauce. Bake for 30 minutes, or until the lasagna is cooked through and the cheese is melted and bubbly.

Chicken served with Cauliflower and Olives

Servings: 2
1 pound chicken breast (boneless, skinless)
1 bunch fresh thyme sprigs
1 head cauliflower, cut into florets
1 shallot, finely chopped
2 tablespoons olive oil
½ teaspoon of sea salt
1 teaspoon ground black pepper
Zest of 1 lemon
¼ cup fresh lemon juice
½ cup Kalamata olives, pitted
2 cloves garlic, thinly sliced

Preheat oven to 400°F. Rinse chicken breasts and pat dry with a paper towel. Spread thyme sprigs evenly in the bottom of a 7 x 11-inch baking dish. Place chicken and cauliflower over the thyme sprigs. In a small bowl, combine shallot, olive oil, salt, pepper, lemon zest and juice, olives and garlic and put the mixture over chicken and cauliflower. Refrigerate for at least one hour or overnight. Bake for 45-55 minutes, until chicken is cooked through, and cauliflower is well browned. Save the other serving for the next day.

Grilled Shrimp and Veggies on a Stick

Servings: 2
1-pound large shrimp, peeled and de-veined
2 tablespoons fresh lemon juice
Sea salt and freshly ground black pepper to taste
1 medium zucchini, sliced into 1" pieces
1 medium yellow summer squash, sliced into 1" pieces
1 red bell pepper, sliced into 2" pieces
1 green bell pepper, sliced into 2" pieces
1 red onion, cut into eighths
2 cloves garlic, minced

3 tablespoons olive oil

Soak wooden skewers in cold water for 30 minutes to prevent burning. Wash and chop vegetables. Prepare grill. In a large bowl, toss together shrimp, lemon juice and pepper. Add vegetables and garlic to the shrimp and add olive oil. Toss. Skewer vegetables and shrimp separately. Place vegetable skewers on the grill and heat on both sides until tender. Place shrimp skewers on the grill and heat until pink on both sides.

Tasty Chicken Marsala with Steamed Broccoli

Servings: 4

¼ cup plus 2 tablespoons olive oil

4 (6 ounce) chicken breasts (boneless, skinless), pounded with meat tenderizer tool

1 cup assorted wild mushrooms, chopped

1 shallot, chopped

½ cup marsala wine

½ cup Cristina's broth (page 106)

½ teaspoon dried oregano

4 cups of fresh broccoli

1 lemon

In a medium pot, steam the broccoli. Add juice of one lemon, ¼ cup of olive oil, and salt and pepper to taste. Set it aside. Heat oil in large skillet over medium heat. Add chicken breasts and cook for 10 minutes, turning at halfway point. Remove from pan and cover. Add mushrooms to pan and cook 5 minutes, stirring occasionally. Stir in shallots and cook one additional minute. Pour in wine and broth, bringing to a boil. Reduce heat and simmer over low heat for 20 minutes. Use a spatula to scrape browned bits from the surface of the pan and mix with liquid. Place chicken back into skillet and cook for five minutes, and sprinkle with oregano. Share it with your family. Serve with broccoli.

Roasted Turkey Breast

Servings: 4
3 tablespoons of olive oil
1 tablespoon of chopped rosemary (fresh or dried)
1 tablespoon of chopped sage (fresh or dried)
1 clove of garlic, minced
2 pounds turkey breast (bone-in, skin on)

Preheat oven to 325°F. Mix olive oil, garlic, sage, and rosemary in a bowl. Rub onto turkey breast. Place turkey breast in a roasting pan, cover with tin foil. Cook for 60 minutes or until internal temperature reaches 165°. After it's cooked, remove from oven, and let it cool for 5 minutes. Carve and enjoy with green beans or vegetables of your choice.

Wild Salmon Basil Burgers

Servings: 4
1 ½ pounds of wild salmon
¼ cup minced fresh basil
1 garlic clove, minced
1 egg
1 teaspoon onion powder (or add minced shallots or onion)
Salt and pepper to taste
Olive oil

Heat large skillet or grill pan to medium heat, or oven to broil. Add oil to pan and allow to heat. Place raw salmon in a food processor with basil and garlic and blend until smooth. Place mixture in a medium bowl. Combine egg, onion, salt, and pepper. Shape into patties and cook for about 7 minutes on each side. You can top with Cristina's Ketchup. Serve with baby arugula drizzled with a squeeze of lemon juice, olive oil, and sprinkled with sea salt and pepper.

Snack Recipes

Cristina's Simple Turkey Protein Dip

Serving Size: 4
1 Pound Ground Turkey
½ Cup Original Cream Cheese
1 Cup Salsa (More or less to taste) - Any Heat Level. Make sure there is no starch or sugar. *Drain liquid from salsa*
Salt and pepper to taste and any other spices you'd like

In a nonstick pan, cook ground turkey and break down. Drain any fat. While still on the heat, mix in cream cheese until totally blended into meat. Drain liquid from salsa. Add salsa. Add salt and pepper to taste. Enjoy ¼ cup of the dip with cut fresh veggies. You may substitute a different meat if you wish, as long as you drain the fat out. Refrigerate/freeze the rest of dip to use when you'd like.

Cristina's Italian Turkey Protein Dip

Serving Size: 4
1 Pound Ground Meat (I used organic ground Turkey)
½ Cup Philadelphia Original Cream Cheese, softened
5-6 scallions, white part, diced
1-2 cloves of garlic, whole or minced
2 big carrots or 3 small carrots, cleaned, diced
3 celery stalks, cleaned, diced
1 big tomato or two small tomatoes, cleaned, diced
½ large cucumber, cleaned, diced
1 jalapeño, cleaned, diced (with or without seeds)
2 cups salsa (optional)
Salt and Pepper to taste
Olive Oil
Fresh cut veggies to dip (Carrots, Celery, Peppers, Cucumbers, etc.)

In a nonstick pan, warm one tablespoon of olive oil. Sauté scallions until almost gold, add garlic, celery, carrots, jalapeño, and salt and pepper. Cook vegetables until soft. Remove from pan and set aside. Cook meat and break it down. Add salt and pepper to taste. Drain any fat. While still on the heat, mix in cream cheese until totally blended into meat. Add sautéed vegetables and remaining diced veggies. Add salsa if you would like. Add salt and pepper to taste. You can serve warm, or you can chill it in the refrigerator for an hour before serving.

Serve as a dip with cut fresh veggies. You can substitute a different meat if you wish, as long as you drain the fat out.

Pepperoni and Cucumber Slices
Serving Size: 1
5 slices pepperoni, unprocessed, no nitrates or preservatives
5 slices cucumber

Cook pepperoni in microwave on paper towel on high for 30 seconds or until crunchy. Serve on top of cucumber and enjoy.

Romaine and Meat Burrito
Serving Size: 1
2 romaine leaves, washed
1-ounce shredded chicken or tuna
Chopped cucumber
Chopped tomatoes
Lemon
Olive oil
Salt, pepper, and spices to taste

Lay leaves out and add ingredients and dress with lemon, olive oil and spices. Roll up with wax paper. Enjoy.

Prosciutto Wrapped Asparagus
Serving Size: 2
4 asparagus stalks, trimmed
¼ tablespoon olive oil
Freshly ground black pepper
4 paper-thin slices prosciutto, halved lengthwise (or thinly sliced ham)

Preheat oven to 400°F. Snap the dry stem ends off of each asparagus and place on a heavy baking sheet. Drizzle with olive oil, sprinkle with pepper, and toss. Roast until the asparagus is tender, about 15 minutes. Cool completely. Wrap each asparagus with 1 piece (about ½ a slice) of prosciutto, exposing tips. Enjoy.

Turkey Bacon and Baked Kale Chips
Serving Size: 1
1 cup of kale leaves
1-2 teaspoons of olive oil
Salt and pepper to taste
2 pieces of turkey bacon, cooked

Preheat oven to 350°F. Toss kale leaves in a bowl with olive oil to coat evenly. On a baking sheet lined with parchment paper lay the leaves flat in a single layer. Pop the tray in the oven, turn the tray after 6 minutes, and after 12 minutes the chips will be done. Once kale is out of the oven, season chips with salt and pepper. Serve immediately with the bacon and enjoy.

Bacon and Goat Cheese Topped Tomato Slices

Serving Size: 1

3 slices of tomato, cut ½ inch thick
2 tablespoons fresh goat cheese
2 teaspoons basil, fresh, chopped
3 pieces bacon, cooked and crumbled
½ teaspoon olive oil

Top tomato slices with goat cheese, basil, and crumbled bacon and drizzle the olive oil on top. Alternatively, broil tomatoes with cheese and basil, until cheese melts, drizzle with olive oil and crumble the bacon on top. Enjoy your healthy snack.

Chicken Yogurt Dip with Veggies

Serving Size: 2

½ cup cooked ground chicken
¼ cup plain yogurt
Sprinkle of seasonings to taste (We chose garlic, onion powder and dried dill)
½ cup mixed raw veggies (baby carrots, cucumber slices, bell peppers, etc.)

Blend chicken and yogurt in your food processor until smooth. Serve ¼ cup of the dip with your ½ cup of veggies. Refrigerate leftover dip.

Beef Jerky

Serving Size: 1

1 ounce of all-natural beef jerky. If you want, this could also be turkey jerky, or any other type of jerky or dried meat you like.

Enjoy with or without a veggie.

Cold Chicken Salad

Serving Size: 1
1½ ounces shredded chicken
½ teaspoon olive oil
Squeeze lemon juice to taste
Salt and pepper to taste
1 tablespoon diced cucumber
1 tablespoon diced celery
1 tablespoon grated carrot
1 lettuce leaf of choice (optional)

Mix together the chicken, veggies, olive oil, lemon juice, and salt and pepper to taste. Serve by itself or wrap into the lettuce leaf if desired.

Shrimp Cocktail

Serving Size: 1
Cocktail sauce (page 107), or any all-natural cocktail sauce with no sugar
2 ounces precooked medium shrimp
2 lettuce leaves (your choice, we chose Boston Bibb)

Dip shrimp in the sauce and enjoy with the lettuce leaves. Include a lemon wedge and fresh parsley to garnish, if desired.

Sliced Chicken and Broccoli

Serving Size: 1
1½ ounces precooked all-natural sliced chicken breast
¼ cup broccoli

Place broccoli in a microwave safe container with ¼ inch of water and heat until broccoli is bright green and tender the way you like it. Season broccoli with salt and pepper and a bit of lemon juice if you wish. Reheat chicken in the microwave until warm.

"BLT"
Serving Size: 1
2 slices precooked turkey bacon, crispy
1 thin slice tomato, cut in half
1 leaf lettuce, torn in strips

Make yourself a mock BLT by stacking the lettuce and tomato alternately and using the turkey bacon for the bread. Enjoy.

Chicken and Spinach Roll Ups
Serving Size: 1
1-ounce thin sliced cooked chicken, uncured, no preservatives
¼ cup fresh baby spinach
2 small yellow bell peppers, chopped

Spread the spinach evenly on each chicken slice. Sprinkle the bell pepper on top. Roll up into the chicken and enjoy.

Turkey with Zucchini Carrot Spread
Serving Size: 3
1-ounce precooked uncured, all-natural turkey cut thinly sliced
2 medium zucchini, cubed
2 carrots, grated
1 small onion, diced
1 teaspoon salt
2 tablespoon olive oil

In a skillet, over medium heat, sauté onions until tender with a small amount of olive oil. Sauté carrots and zucchini until tender. Add salt and spice of your choice and mix well. Remove from heat and let cool. In a food processor puree zucchini-carrot mixture. Make your zucchini spread in the morning and take 1/3 of it with you for your snack. Spread your turkey slices with the zucchini and roll up if desired. Enjoy and save the leftovers.

Tuna with Baby Spinach and Cherry Tomatoes

Serving Size: 1

1 ounce tuna, all natural, canned
½ cup baby spinach
3 cherry tomatoes cut in half
1 lemon wedge for juice
1 teaspoon olive oil

Create a little salad with tuna, spinach, and tomatoes for yourself. Squeeze lemon over it to taste, and drizzle olive oil. Enjoy

Turkey Jerky

Serving Size: 1

½ ounce of all-natural turkey jerky. You can have this with any veggie of choice or by itself if you prefer.

Chicken and Shredded Carrots

Serving Size: 1

1-ounce cooked chicken breast
¼ cup shredded carrots (or another shredded veggie)

Heat chicken in the microwave and serve over your raw shredded carrots. You may also heat carrots in the microwave with a bit of water to steam. Enjoy.

Turkey Bacon Roll Ups

Serving Size: 1

1 ounce turkey bacon, cooked
2 romaine lettuce leaves
1 slice fresh mozzarella
2 cherry tomatoes, halved

In each romaine leaf place a slice of turkey bacon, followed by half a slice of mozzarella cheese, and 2 halves each of cherry tomatoes. Roll up the leaf and enjoy.

Shrimp Salad with Broccoli
Serving Size: 1
2 ounces salad shrimp, precooked
¼ cup cooked broccoli
Lemon wedge for juice
Salt and pepper to taste

Heat the shrimp and broccoli in the microwave together for one minute, or until warm. Sprinkle shrimp and broccoli with lemon juice and salt and pepper to taste if you would like.

Shrimp and Corn Salad
Serving Size: 1
2 ounces salad shrimp, precooked
¼ cup cooked corn, cooled
2 cherry tomatoes, halved
2 slices cucumber, halved

Heat up your shrimp if you want it warm. Mix together the corn, tomatoes, and cucumber. Top with the shrimp and enjoy.

Mini Tuna Bites with Cucumber
Serving Size: 1
6 thin slices cucumber
2-ounce shredded tuna from can or package, no preservatives
Celery (chopped)
Squeeze lemon juice
Drizzle olive oil
Salt, pepper, and spices to taste

Mix tuna with the other ingredients to create a salad consistency. Split up evenly and top three of your cucumber slices with the tuna salad. Add the additional cucumber slices to create three mini sandwiches. Enjoy.

Turkey Bacon and Cucumber Slices
Serving Size: 1
2 pieces turkey bacon
4-5 cucumber slices

Enjoy together. Heat turkey bacon in the microwave for two minutes on high or until crispy, depending on the power of your microwave.

Sliced Turkey with Veggies
Serving Size: 1
1½ ounces sliced cooked turkey
Handful fresh baby spinach
Mini bell pepper, chopped
3 cherry tomatoes, halved
1 lemon wedge for juice
½ tablespoon olive oil
Salt and pepper to taste

Combine spinach, pepper, and cherry tomatoes in a small bowl. Squeeze lemon and drizzle your olive oil. Sprinkle salt and pepper to taste. Top with the sliced turkey and enjoy.

Chicken Salad with Avocado
Serving Size: 1
1 teaspoon avocado
Juice of a lemon wedge
1 teaspoon celery, chopped small
1 teaspoon cucumber, diced
½ teaspoon onion powder
2 ounce cooked shredded chicken, not canned
Sea salt and pepper to taste

Mix avocado, chicken, lemon juice, celery, onion powder, and salt and pepper to taste in a small bowl with a fork. Enjoy.

Miscellaneous Recipes

Cristina's Cauliflower Rice
Servings: 4
1 head cauliflower, washed, trimmed, and separated into florets

To make the cauliflower rice, pulse batches of raw cauliflower florets in a food processor until a rice-like texture is achieved. You can cook as you normally would with rice.

Cristina's Chicken and Beef Broth
Servings: Dependent on time left reducing
4 Beef bones
1 chicken (raw chicken, well washed)
3 carrots
3 celery stalks with leaves
4 scallions (remove greens)
3 Fresh tomatoes (cut and seeded) or 3 canned whole tomatoes (with no seeds and no citric acid)

Fill a big pot with cold water. Wash all meat and add to the water. Bring to a boil. Begin to skim the fat and waste off the top when you see it. Simmer and skim until there is no more fat and waste. Clean carrots, celery, scallions, and tomatoes and add to broth. Let simmer for 5-7 hours until bones separate from meat. Use tongs to remove bones and a strainer to remove vegetables from broth. Let cool and skim off the excess fat when it is cold. Add salt and pepper to taste.

To Make Soup:
Add meat (ground turkey, pork, beef, or chicken – cooked and grease drained)
Add vegetables (such as zucchini, green beans, carrots, escarole, spinach, kale)
Use equal amount of meat and vegetables and cut small.

Cristina's Ketchup
Servings: 4
2 tablespoons olive oil
6 scallions (cleaned, only the white part, not the green)
5 ripe medium tomatoes
Salt and pepper to taste and any other spices you'd like

In a nonstick pan, warm 2 tablespoons of olive oil. Take the 6 scallions (white part) and chop them into small pieces and add to warm oil. Let caramelize without burning on low heat. In a separate pot, boil enough water to cover your 5 tomatoes. Add tomatoes once the water is boiling. Within 2 to 3 minutes, tomatoes will be ready to peel and seed. When they cool, chop into small pieces, and add to the caramelized scallions. At this time, you can add the salt, pepper, and spices if you wish. Let this cook over low heat until it becomes the consistency of ketchup or desired consistency. If you prefer to have a smoother ketchup, you can use your blender to reach that consistency.

You can multiply this recipe if you wish. If you do not have scallions, you may substitute sweet onions. If you do not have ripe tomatoes, you can substitute peeled canned tomatoes as long as they do not have citric acid. Drain and seed canned tomatoes first.

*To make **BBQ Sauce**, add desired spices and a few drops of honey*

Cristina's Cocktail Sauce
Servings: 4
2 cups Cristina's ketchup (page 107)
1 teaspoon Worcestershire sauce
1 teaspoon lemon juice
Zest from half a lemon
2 tablespoons fresh grated horseradish

Mix and chill for one hour.

Cristina's Meatballs without Bread

Servings: 5
1 lb. ground beef (leanest you can find)
½ lb. ground veal
½ lb. ground pork
2 eggs, lightly beaten
½ cup grated Parmigiano-Reggiano cheese
½ cup grated Pecorino cheese (If you cannot find or do not have, you can use 1 cup Parmigiano-Reggiano instead)
¼ cup finely chopped fresh flat-leaf parsley
1 garlic clove, minced (optional)
Salt and pepper to taste
1 tablespoon water
Optional: 2 small zucchinis grated. Do not use the tablespoon of water if you use the zucchini.
Cristina's sauce (made ahead of time) (page 109)

Preheat oven to 375°F. In a large bowl, combine the beef, veal, pork, eggs, cheese, parsley, garlic, salt, and a few grinds of pepper. Add the zucchini to the meat mixture and mix gently until combined. Rinse your hands with water but do not dry them. Shape the meat into 2-inch balls, rolling them lightly between your moistened palms. In a 13x9 inch pan with sides, add enough boiling water to go halfway up the meatballs. Drop meatballs in. The water will keep the meatballs with a soft consistency. Bake in oven no more than 7 to 10 minutes until the outside is cooked and the inside is still a little red. All the fat will go into the water. Drop the meatballs into the sauce made ahead of time and let cook for 45 minutes to 1 hour. You can freeze the meatballs, but please freeze them separately from the sauce.

Cristina's Sauce

Servings: 5

3 – 24-ounce cans of organic tomatoes or San Marzano without citric acid or salt
3 or 4 beef ribs, cut
2 pork chops
3 tablespoons olive oil
1 small onion or the white part of three scallions
1 carrot, cleaned, cut in half.
1 celery stalk, cleaned, cut in half
Salt and pepper

Do not use an aluminum pot. Use nonstick or porcelain. Blend tomatoes in blender. Sauté onion or scallion, carrot, and celery with olive oil on low heat to caramelize them. Remove from pot and set aside. Using the same pan, cook the meat on both sides until well done. Add the tomatoes, vegetables that have been set aside, and salt and pepper to the pot. Let sauce simmer for hours until it reaches the texture you want and until the meat separates from the bone. With a slotted spoon - remove bones, meat, and vegetables. Skim the fat off the top. You now have a clean sauce.

Nut-Free Basil Pesto

Servings: 6

4 cups fresh basil, trimmed
Juice of half a lemon
1 clove garlic, peeled
¼ cup olive oil
2 tablespoons Parmigiano-Reggiano
Salt and pepper to taste
(You may add ¼ cup of pine nuts or any other nuts you would like)

Purée all ingredients in your food processor until desired texture. Place in container and refrigerate.

Cristina's Mashed Cauliflower
Servings: 4
1 pound cauliflower, washed, trimmed, and separated into florets
¼ cup Cristina's broth (page 106) or milk/cream
¼ cup grated Parmigiano-Reggiano
Salt and pepper

Steam or cook cauliflower in microwave. Do not cook in water.
Add to blender with salt, pepper, grated Parmigiano-Reggiano and
broth or milk/cream until it reached the consistency that you like.

Cristina's Spaghetti Squash
Cut the spaghetti squash in half lengthwise. Remove seeds and
pulp from one half.
Microwave: Microwave squash on high for 8 minutes or less, then
use a fork to loosen squash from the skin and scrape the strands
into a bowl.
Oven: Preheat the oven to 375°F. Place both halves face down on a
baking pan, with ¼" of water. Bake for 45 minutes. Dig out squash
with a fork (crosswise) and scrape strands into a bowl.

Cristina's Chicken Cacciatore
Servings: 3
6 chicken thighs bone in, skin on, trimmed of excess fat
Salt and black pepper
Extra virgin olive oil
1 small yellow onion, chopped
2 celery ribs, chopped
½ red bell pepper, chopped
½ green bell pepper, chopped
8 ounces mushrooms (white or baby Bella) cleaned and sliced
3 garlic cloves, minced

1 teaspoon oregano
3 sprigs fresh thyme
2 tablespoon fresh chopped parsley, more for later
Pinch red pepper flakes
1 cup red wine
28 ounce can crushed tomatoes, without citric acid

Pat the chicken dry and season with salt and pepper on both sides and underneath the skin. In a large pan or braiser (with a lid), heat 2 tablespoons of extra-virgin olive oil over medium-high until simmering but not smoking. Add the chicken, skin side down first. Cook until golden brown, then turn over to brown on the other side (about 8 minutes total). Remove the chicken and set aside on a plate. In the same braiser, add the onions, celery, peppers, mushrooms, and garlic. Cook over medium heat, tossing regularly. Add salt, pepper, oregano, fresh thyme, parsley, and red pepper flakes. Allow the vegetables to cook for 5 to 6 minutes or until tender. Add the red wine and cook for a few minutes until the wine has reduced by about ½, then add the tomatoes. Cook 5 to 10 minutes over medium heat, stirring occasionally. Now add the chicken pieces back to the pan. Reduce the heat to medium-low. Cover and allow the chicken to cook for 30 minutes or until cooked through. Garnish with parsley.

Cristina's Slow Cooker Pulled Pork
Servings: 6
5–7-pound pork butt or pork shoulder leave the fat cap on
3 tablespoons olive oil for rubbing on meat
1 tablespoon olive oil
1 tablespoon kosher salt use 2 and 1/2 teaspoons if using table salt
2 teaspoons black pepper
1 tablespoon paprika

2 teaspoons garlic powder
2 teaspoons onion powder
1 teaspoon chili powder
1 teaspoon cayenne pepper
2 teaspoons cumin
1 teaspoon dry mustard powder
1 tablespoon brown sugar
2 medium carrots, chopped
2 celery stalks, chopped
1 medium onion, chopped
4oz red or white wine
1-2 cups Cristina's BBQ Sauce (page 107)

In a small bowl, combine 1 tablespoon kosher salt, 2 teaspoons black pepper, 1 tablespoon paprika, 2 teaspoons garlic powder, 2 teaspoons onion powder, 1 teaspoon chili powder, 1 teaspoon cayenne pepper, 2 teaspoon cumin, 1 teaspoon dry mustard powder and brown sugar. Split in half and reserve for later. Use paper towels to dry off the pork as best you can. Massage 1 tablespoon olive oil into the meat, making sure it's well distributed. Use your hands to rub the spices into the meat, getting every nook and cranny and under every flap. Place in a large zip lock bag and seal. Marinate in the fridge for at least 6 hours, or up to 48 hours. Remove the pork from the zip lock and pat dry if it is wet. Rub the remaining spice rub mixture into the pork. Set a large dry skillet on your stove over medium high heat. Let the skillet preheat for at least 3 minutes on medium high. Add a drizzle of olive oil and swirl to coat the pan. Add the pork and sear for about 2 minutes until well browned. Use tongs to flip the pork and sear the other side until browned. Flip again onto its side, until all the outside of the pork is seared. Place the seared pork into your dry crock pot.

Add wine to deglaze pan and then add celery, carrots and onion and sauté them until tender. Add your pork. Cover with the lid and cook on low heat for about 8-10 hours, turning occasionally. In the last hour, add Cristina's BBQ Sauce. Shred the pork using two forks. Remove any gristle. Enjoy with spaghetti squash or spiralized zucchini.

Gelato (Maintenance Only)
Servings: 4
2 cups milk
1 cup heavy cream
4 egg yolks
1 cup fruit – sweet – cut into pieces

In a medium saucepan, mix milk and cream. Warm until foam forms around the edges. Remove from heat. In a large bowl, beat the egg yolks until frothy. Gradually pour the warm milk into the egg yolks, whisking constantly. Return mixture to saucepan; cook over medium heat, stirring with a wooden spoon until the mixture gels slightly and coats the back of the spoon. If small egg lumps begin to show, remove from heat immediately. Pour the mixture through a sieve or fine strainer into a bowl. Mix in fruit. Cover, and chill for several hours or overnight. Pour the mixture into an ice cream maker and freeze according to the manufacturer's instructions. Transfer to a sealed container and freeze until firm. If the gelato is too firm, place it in the refrigerator until it reaches the desired consistency.

Glossary of Terms

Healthy Lifestyle:

To achieve a healthy lifestyle is to have a good nutritional intake, daily exercise, adequate sleep, and positive sense of self, as well as stress management.

Natural foods:

Natural food is food that has not been altered in any way.

Wholesome:

Wholesome means promoting anything that is healthy emotionally, physically, or spiritually.

Spiralize:

To spiralize the vegetables you can choose from a few different methods. A spiralizer is a device you can buy from any home goods store nearby. If you don't have one or want to get one a julienne blade attached to your regular vegetable peeler works almost as well. And an alternative to that method would be to simply grate or slice the vegetables thinly.

Bibliography:

Sisson, Mark. *The Primal Blueprint.* Malibu, CA: Primal Nutrition, 2009. Print.
Davis, William. *La Dieta Zero Grano.* New York, NY: Rodale Books, 2011. Print.

Index of Recipes

Breakfast Recipes

Salads

Chicken and Kale Salad, 64

Tuna Topped Spinach Salad, 62

Simply Chicken Spinach Salad, 69

Beef & Lamb Dishes

Beef and Butternut Squash Stew, 69

Lamb with Sweet Red Peppers, 74

Scrumptious Spanish Spaghetti
Squash with Olives, 87

Spaghetti with Meatballs, 88

Healthy Shepherd's Pie (Beef), 89

Cristina's Meatballs without Bread,
108

Pork Dishes

Italian Sausage Mushroom Caps, 70

Healthy Pizza with Homemade
Cauliflower Crust, 74

Crock Pot Pork Loin, 75

Baked Italian-Style Portabella
Mushrooms with Prosciutto and
Mozzarella, 78

Cristina's Stuffed Turkey Eggplant
Rollatini, 82

Eggplant Lasagna, 91

Cristina's Slow Cooker Pulled Pork,
111

Poultry Dishes

Simply Chicken Spinach Salad, 69

Cristina's Turkey Burgers with
Grated Zucchini and Carrots, 70

Tasty Chicken Cutlet Sandwich, 72

Spaghetti Squash with Pesto, 72

Rustic Breadless Chicken with
Artichokes, 76

Turkey and Veggie Fajitas, 78

Cristina's Stuffed Turkey Eggplant
Rollatini, 82

Classic Chicken Parmesan, 83

Tangy Salsa Chicken, 85

Healthy Shepherd's Pie (Turkey or
Chicken), 89

Stuffed Peppers with Ground
Chicken, 86

Grilled Chicken with Lemon and
Rosemary, 88

Chicken Nuggets with Carrot, 90

Chicken served with Cauliflower
and Olives, 92

Tasty Chicken Marsala with
Steamed Broccoli, 93

Roasted Turkey Breast, 94

Cristina's Chicken Cacciatore, 110

Seafood Dishes

Endive Salmon Poppers, 71

Peppercorn Tuna Skewers with Eggplant, 71
Delightful Salmon with Garlic, Spinach, and Tomatoes, 73
Red Snapper Scampi with Steamed Veggies, 73
Mediterranean-Style Tuna with Garlic, Parsley, and Tomatoes, 76

Traditional Italian Fish Stew, 77
Slow-Cooked Spanish Cod, 84
Scallops and Asparagus Entrée, 85
Grilled Shrimp and Veggies on a Stick, 92
Wild Salmon Basil Burgers, 94

Share with your Family

Cristina's Classic Frittata with Veggies, 58
Beef and Butternut Squash Stew, 69
Cristina's Turkey Burgers with Grated Zucchini and Carrots, 70
Delightful Salmon with Garlic, Spinach, and Tomatoes, 73
Healthy Pizza with Homemade Cauliflower Crust, 74
Crock Pot Pork Loin, 75
Cristina's Stuffed Turkey Eggplant Rollatini, 82

Tangy Salsa Chicken, 85
Spaghetti with Meatballs, 88
Eggplant Lasagna, 91
Tasty Chicken Marsala with Steamed Broccoli, 93
Roasted Turkey Breast, 94
Wild Salmon Basil Burgers, 94
Cristina's Chicken Cacciatore, 110
Cristina's Slow Cooker Pulled Pork, 111

Italian Classics

Cristina's Classic Frittata with Veggies, 58
Healthy Pizza with Homemade Cauliflower Crust, 74
Cristina's Stuffed Turkey Eggplant Rollatini, 82

Classic Chicken Parmesan, 83
Eggplant Lasagna, 91
Cristina's Meatballs without Bread, 108
Cristina's Chicken Cacciatore, 110

Snacks & Miscellaneous

Cristina's Turkey Protein Dip – two ways, 96
Pepperoni and Cucumber Slices, 97
Romaine and Meat Burrito, 97

Prosciutto wrapped Asparagus, 98
Turkey Bacon and Baked Kale Chips, 98